MOMMYSATTVA

MOMMYSATTVA

CONTEMPLATIONS FOR
MOTHERS WHO MEDITATE
(OR WISH THEY COULD)

Jenna Hollenstein

The information in this volume is not intended as a substitute
for consultation with health care professionals. Each individual's
health concerns should be evaluated by a qualified professional.

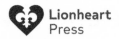

Lionheart Press, Somerville, MA, USA
lionheartpress.net

Library of Congress Control Number: 2021909459

ISBN 978-1-7322776-6-3 (paperback)
ISBN 978-1-7322776-7-0 (e-book)

Cover design by Alex Hennig (fleck creative studio)
Interior design by Jazmin Welch (fleck creative studio)
Interior illustrations courtesy of Grace Li (mazehandmade.com)

Dedicated to the members of the
Open Heart Project Mommy Sangha—
past, present, and future

CONTENTS

INTRODUCTION • 1

MATRESCENCE • 17

MEDITATION • 73

MOTHERHOOD IS THE PATH • 107

THE MOTHER'S BODY • 163

EVERY CHILD IS A BUDDHA • 185

MOTHERS AS SOCIAL JUSTICE • 213

THE FIERCE MOTHER LINEAGE • 235

Acknowledgments • 247

About the Author • 249

INTRODUCTION

IT IS 5:30 ON A TUESDAY MORNING, five months into the 2020 coronavirus pandemic, and I am up to start putting together these thoughts. Pre-motherhood, I was not a morning person, but now, when else do I have the time, space, and mental real estate to do such a thing? My five-year-old son will be up within the hour, and my attention will be diverted from reflection to more immediate needs like breakfast, reminders to pee, and negotiating activities other than playing video games (on which I have relied heavily during this period and which may very well have contributed to a new facial tic I noticed in him a couple of weeks ago).

Once schools were shuttered, his pre-K class time consisted of a mere 15-minute virtual morning meeting—no fault of the teachers—followed by a series of "optional" activities, or in other words, homework for the parents, mostly moms. Everywhere, moms scrambled to deal with the rapid shift in expectations. Then summer officially started after his "moving-up" ceremony with most camps canceled and other summer activities not an option. Our flight to Sicily to visit my partner's family—that delightful annual respite of sea and cousins and childcare carried out by persons other than me—was out of the question. My

1

partner was back to work full time at a research institute, so if not for the pathological helpfulness of my parents I would have had to stop seeing clients or (*shudder*) work in the evenings when my brain and body have used up all their capacity and I am counting the minutes until bedtime.

Our newfound "freedom" from our plans leaves us at loose ends. We try to get outside—a challenge in New York City due to the congestion and the summer swelter. We try to see other kids—complicated by the refrain of "Six feet!" and dissolution of social skills from five months of homeschooling. We try to do some form of learning—practicing writing his name, reading Mo Willems, journaling the progress of his expensive butterfly habitat, adding and subtracting gummy bears, playing sight word bingo. Usually we just get through the day and I try not to feel too badly about it.

We spend a lot of time together. He's growing in front of my eyes. I know this because my eyes are on him every waking moment. More than my eyes—my entire body is attuned to his throughout the day. I'm constantly sensing his moods. Is this sadness, anger, exhaustion, hypoglycemia? Is it the irritable perfectionism he inherited from me (god help him)? I navigate the fine line between relieving his discomfort and helping him learn to deal with it himself.

My body is his home base. My eyes must witness his invention of a new dance move or when he puts on slippery socks and "speed skates" in the living room like Frozone from *The Incredibles*. My ears and mouth must hear and affirm when he discovers what N-E-S-T spells or unlocks a new Marvel video game character. "Yes!," "Yes?," and "I'm listening" are repeated hundreds of times each day. If my body disappears behind the bathroom door, it isn't for long. My body is the most powerful instrument I own, the constant that communicates with presence and touch and reciprocity that I am here for him no matter what, that my love for him only grows, even—or especially—in difficulty.

When he wakes, he'll come in for a quick cuddle and then sit alongside me, watching "Pencilmation" on his iPad but needing the reassurance of my body nearby. At this point I'll abandon my laptop, the sanctity of this space and time interrupted until tomorrow morning before we begin our day all over again. (Harold Ramis, wherever you are, it's time for a remake of *Groundhog Day* from a mom's perspective.)

This squeeze of time and space replicated in households all over the globe makes it nearly impossible for mothers to recognize, reflect on, value, and share the work they are doing, let alone convey that value to the world. Knowing every other mother on the planet is going through some form of this right now provides little comfort. The monolith, Motherhood, is heralded by many as the hardest job in the world, yet the lack of systemic support for mothers—scanty maternity leave (in the United States and other mostly non-EU countries around the world), lack of affordable childcare, few broadly accessible mental health resources, limited supportive communities, inconsistently supportive partners, rare candid discussions of the challenges faced by mothers, zero safety net in the case of, say, a global pandemic—says otherwise.

This strange time has shone a spotlight on the attitude we hold toward motherhood, reflected in *The New York Times* articles such as "In the COVID-19 Economy, You Can Have a Kid or a Job. You Can't Have Both," "America's Mothers Are in Crisis," and "How Society Has Turned Its Back on Mothers." We've forwarded these articles to one another in the wee hours of the morning, but they haven't sparked a national debate (let alone action) about whether this state of existence is just, sustainable, or humane. Anyone invested in having that debate was too exhausted to engage in it anyway. The disconnect between our own awareness of the true importance of motherhood and the capacity to change how it is regarded in the larger culture makes motherhood something we largely experience alone. Long before the order to shelter in place, moms were already isolated, individually doing the mental math of how to work and parent and take care of all the things in a focused, present, worthwhile way, often feeling judged by one another and perhaps even more harshly by ourselves.

As a practicing Buddhist and meditator of more than thirteen years, the lens through which I view my own life and our interconnected lives is one of ordinary sacredness, of energies in flux, and of infinite opportunities to experience enlightenment in everyday life. I did not arrive at this view through conceptual understanding—although I appreciate intellect very much. I realized this through experiencing the movement of my mind as my body sat in stillness. That act alone, though shockingly difficult, has been alongside motherhood the most instructive arc of my life. As a result, I strongly feel the cognitive dissonance of our personal and collective imbalance, confusion, and crisis.

In *Wisdom Rising: Journey into the Mandala of the Empowered Feminine*, Lama Tsultrim Allione writes:

> The loss of feminine qualities is an urgent psychological and ecological issue in modern society. It is a painful loss in our emotional lives and a disastrous loss for the safety of life on earth. In woman, it affects her central identity; and in man, it affects his ability to feel and value. The loss of the feminine in man causes him to feel moody and lonely. In woman, it causes her to lose faith in herself. We are slowly awakening to the crisis of the earth and the effect of the

loss of the sacred feminine, but few people understand that the causes of the crisis have spiritual values at their roots— values of the sacred as immanent, imbued in all of life, and all life as interdependent.

The Buddhist view of feminine and masculine is concerned with energies, not to be confused with gender and how its constructs have come into being in our current culture. Just as we all possess a left brain hemisphere and a right brain hemisphere, we all possess feminine and masculine energies. Both as individuals and as a collective society, feminine and masculine energies are expressed in ways that can contribute to balance or imbalance, wisdom or confusion. As Lama Tsultrim states, and as I have observed as a mother in a culture that does not seem to have my back, we are in a chronic state of imbalance and confusion.

In Buddhism, especially Tantric Buddhism, a harmonious balance of masculine and feminine qualities is necessary to realize enlightenment. The Buddha is very often represented as having a perfect balance of the masculine and feminine. Although we know that the representations are of a man-bodied person, if we did not know this, we might well think them images of a woman. This is very much on purpose as an illustrative metaphor of masculine and feminine. How these qualities unfold and express themselves in the individual and in the environment is the true foundation for waking up to reality.

During quarantine, my partner taught himself how to play the piano. Granted, his brain works differently than most, and he becomes a dog with a bone whenever something is challenging and interesting. Five months in and he is playing Chopin, Pachelbel, and Handel. He has this newly acquired skill, this bucket list accomplishment, to show for the months in isolation.

The pieces he plays have come to serve as the soundtrack for my loading and unloading the dishwasher, folding the laundry, chopping garlic and onions.

It would be easy to feel aggrieved: he gets to learn and practice a glorified skill while I have to look after all those less glorified and more mundane tasks around the house. (Before you hate him too much, know that he works his butt off, pays all our bills, cooks half the time, and is the chief IT officer and travel agent in our household.) And at the same time, I deeply enjoy doing these everyday tasks. They are not the only things I do in a day, but these quotidian duties are the glue that holds it all together. I take pride in cooking for my family, cleaning up the apartment, even doing the laundry (though I'd give anything to have a washer and dryer in the apartment instead of in the basement of our building). I just wish, however, that they occupied the same overall value as piano playing. In our productivity-obsessed culture, I have wondered, "Do I have something to show for my time in quarantine?" The answer I keep coming back to is "That is the wrong question."

So what is the right question? It has something to do with whether and how we met the challenges of having the rug pulled out from under us again and again. It is related to our capacity to open to uncertainty and change—and how we modeled that for our kids—rather than clamping down on some sort of project or self-improvement scheme to distract us from the reality of the difficulties. I'm fairly certain the right questions include "Were you there for it—the uncertainty, the discomfort, the groundlessness? Did you show up? Did you stay with it? Did you allow yourself to feel?"

Even if we personally value and derive satisfaction from whatever tasks we routinely engage in, domestic and otherwise, it matters that the larger society does not. We feel deep internal conflicts for doing the work that is viewed as menial while loftier accomplishments are prized. Or we feel the need to absorb those tasks into an even grander scheme of "doing it all" and "having it all." In the words of Michelle Obama, "That shit doesn't work." Even if we enjoy these undertakings, we can harbor resentment if we have not been given a choice about doing them, if no one else is contributing, and, for me especially, if they remain invisible and unappreciated.

A mother's version of the classic John Lennon song might be "Imagine there's no wage gap / It isn't hard to do." But, seriously, imagine if women were paid equitably for their work inside and outside the home. Imagine if employment benefits packages included daycare and after-school care. Imagine if hospitals and midwives handed off new mothers to the care of outpatient mental health support systems with regular check-ins. What would life be like if support groups for mothers were as plentiful, varied, and ordinary as Alcoholics Anonymous meetings—those for moms of kids with special needs, foster moms, adoptive moms, stepmoms, moms attempting to blend families with wisdom and compassion? What if mom guilt was a thing of the past, and what if in response to rare relapses regarding prioritizing convenience in meal prep, delegating housecleaning to family members or a paid employee, or forgetting School Pajama Day, everyone invoked the now well-known phrase "Momma, you're good"? Call me a dreamer, but I'm not the only one.

It would be easy to internalize society's value system in which the grit and monotony of motherhood is seen as lesser. Whether stay-at-home moms (SAHMs), mompreneurs, moms who work outside the home, moms seeking work at a living wage, or moms who are in transition between any of the above, we face an often unwinnable battle for feelings of accomplishment, productivity, and usefulness. But suppose we flipped the script? Rather than it being the number of widgets sold, emails sent, or papers pushed, or the appearance of being "Instafabulous" and showing the world how you are rocking it, imagine if we chose to prioritize moments of presence, gentleness, and compassion.

There is a vast chasm between how we experience motherhood internally and how it is regarded externally. To collectively view motherhood as of the utmost importance would require a complete renovation of our principles and ideologies. A smashing of the capitalist patriarchal system to value presence as highly as productivity, kindness and compassion as highly as dollars and cents. A dismantling of the oversimplified hierarchy that places SAHMS on one rung of a ladder and the working supermom on another. A view that goes beyond the rigged game encouraging moms to accept themselves as "good enough" while simultaneously inventing unattainable mom goals and selling distractions disguised as self-care. One that celebrates mothers in all their rage and joy and grief and ecstasy. That venerates the mother's body for its astounding physical and emotional capacities and the succor it provides, rather than reducing it to a superficial object to aspire to, fix, or camouflage.

A mother has a vested interest in the world being a more compassionate, cooperative, and sane place to live. She has no choice but to take an interest in leaving the world better than she found it for those in her care. So not only does the mother commit to devoting her life to the benefit of her own children, she must also be thinking bigger; she must be ever widening the circle of her compassion.

WHO IS A MOMMYSATTVA?

THIS BOOK IS AN ODE TO THE PATH of enlightenment that is motherhood. Individuals who dedicate their lives to being of benefit to others are known as *bodhisattvas*. They vow to work with their own minds to develop wisdom and compassion but delay their own enlightenment out of the knowledge of our interconnectedness with all living beings. Whether or not she intends to, and regardless of whether or not she's Buddhist, a woman who becomes a mother takes the vow to be of benefit to others. She becomes a "mommysattva": a warrior of compassion, wisdom, and lovingkindness.

Inherent to the mommysattva is an expansive definition of "Mother." A mother is the woman who gives birth to her child. A mother is the woman who adopts a child she has not birthed, becomes a child's stepmother, or fosters a child. A mother may be a grandmother, father, older sibling, or another relative. A mother may be someone outside the traditional family circle with whom a mother–child bond is clear. A mother may be chosen by the child. She is the default caregiver, the primary influence in a child's life, their North Star. She is the one who takes ultimate responsibility for the child and does whatever is necessary for their care. Ultimately, a mother—the one who mothers—is the center of the mandala.

A mandala is a geometric shape, usually a circle (it is the Sanskrit word for "circle"), that is used to demonstrate the organization of an entity and how and where the various pieces of that entity fit together. It is an image ultimately of the relationship between different parts of a whole. The mandala was a source of inspiration for Carl Jung, who believed that it provided a visual and mental tool to discover the authentic self. By moving from the outer circle toward its center, individuals could discern the true self from the illusory one. In Buddhism, mandalas are used to tell the stories of individuals, such as the Buddha or various bodhisattvas, or the stories of central themes, such as the nature of suffering. Always at the center is the person or entity from which all else arises.

In the summer of 2020, during a rare escape from the city to my parents on Long Island, I was finally able to get into the ocean and look out over the water. When I turned back to the beach and saw all the beachgoers playing in the waves and on the shore, I was deeply struck by the fact that each and every one of these bodies originated in the belly of a woman. That they entered the world by being pushed out through a vagina or lifted directly out of a uterus. That each body was cared for by that originator or someone else who stepped into the role. Mothers create the world and those who mother tend to its inhabitants.

The weight of the mother–child relationship—its presence or absence, how it underlies the way we speak to ourselves, how we love others, build relationships, navigate difficulty—cannot be overstated. It is deeply connected to the narratives we carry with us for the rest of our lives. It is the vast constellation of seemingly infinitesimal moments in which mothers guide, validate, nurture, and are present for their children, which in turn influences who they ultimately become and how they contribute to the world. A mother's attention, attunement, patience, steadfastness, and grace (for herself and others) communicate to her children that they are good, worthy, and deserving of unconditional love and com-passion. In this way—sometimes quietly, other times loudly—mothers create the world. The role of the mother is foundational. Determinational. Sacred.

With the role of mother so universal and so integral to the mental and physical well-being of the Earth's inhabitants, and if so many of us are experiencing the same struggles, why do we continue to feel isolated, undervalued, and unseen? Why do we not recognize motherhood as the transformational path to awakening that it is and connect with other mothers as divine and powerful sisters?

The solution lies in recognizing the mommysattva. She understands the full importance of the responsibility she has assumed. She is invested in working with her own confusion, uncertainty, and difficulty. She craves realness, wishes to discover the nature of reality, desires to get to the heart of the matter, and is not afraid of the struggle, pain, and true joy required to do so.

WHAT IS THE MOMMY SANGHA?

THE OPEN HEART PROJECT MOMMY SANGHA was founded in 2016 and has met every single week with few exceptions. Moms of all backgrounds and from all over log into Zoom to practice meditation together for a few minutes, reflect on the Buddha's teachings as they relate to motherhood, connect, and share a space in which motherhood is regarded as sacred.

Founding and leading the Mommy Sangha has shaped my understanding of motherhood as a path and practice. Week after week, together we have realized how our experiences as mothers reflect the most basic questions inherent in being human: about happiness and suffering, how to work with difficulty, issues around being versus doing, learning to accept our lives as they unfold, finding stability and joy in the midst of our messy, imperfect lives. We have realized how in narrowing our focus to a single point—whether in feeling the breath in meditation practice or in the laser-sharp attention we pay to our children's cries—our connection to all beings actually expands.

When the pandemic hit, I was relieved that the Mommy Sangha already existed. Many of us with school-age kids felt as if we were back in the newborn stage of motherhood: tethered to the home, our mobility suddenly dramatically restricted, isolated from one another without access to our usual coping strategies. Some mothers of children with special needs felt that others were experiencing what was their norm before the pandemic. Within the community of the Mommy Sangha, we were able to explore how the pandemic magnified a lot of the issues we had already identified in motherhood.

As it turns out, the pandemic provided an ideal testing– practice–training ground for the mommysattva. How we experienced the coronavirus pandemic was hugely impacted by the fact that we are mothers. Our lives slowed down. Dynamics between ourselves and our partners, kids, and other family members intensified. Our patience was tested again and again, our plans upended, and our attachments disrupted. Uncertainty flourished. A lot of this was painful and at the same time illuminating. We got to see ourselves reacting to the big squeeze between our hopes and fears, our expectations and reality.

Throughout the pandemic, the Mommy Sangha practiced together. We celebrated new pregnancies, supported one another through moves, illness, job changes, and divorce, laughed together about the shocking words that come out of our kids' mouths, and solidified our commitment to keep showing up for ourselves and one another—literally and figuratively. The opportunity to sit together, to hold space for one another, to laugh and cry and breathe together has been a lifeline that preceded the pandemic, endured throughout, and I hope will continue in one form or another well into the future. I am so grateful to these women for enriching this book and my life in general. I invite you, through this book, to feel part of this community.

ENGAGING THIS BOOK

THE SHORT PASSAGES THAT MAKE UP THIS BOOK speak to the momentous spiritual importance of even the smallest interactions between ourselves and our children and, perhaps even more importantly, between ourselves and ourselves. We acknowledge the critical spiritual significance of mothers, beginning by first recognizing this in ourselves, then seeing it in one another, and finally sharing this understanding with the world.

The book is divided into seven sections. In the first section, "Matrescence," the Buddhist and Western psychological worlds collide, and together we look at the transformed identity of the mother and how this rarely discussed metamorphosis and its attendant emotional rollercoaster rocks us to the core and has aftershocks that last the rest of our days.

In "Meditation," I provide the simplest instructions I know of for working with our minds and ask critical questions (and perhaps even discover a few answers) about how to hold our minds and hearts on the path to enlightenment.

"Motherhood Is the Path" touches on the countless ways in which the path of motherhood is inextricable from the path to enlightenment; the passages are intended to serve as reminders of the endless intersections between Buddhist philosophy and what we encounter every day as mothers.

"The Mother's Body" acknowledges the wonder of these vessels we walk around in, introducing a fresh way of relating to this instrument that largely determines how we show up in our children's lives as well as our own.

"Every Child Is a Buddha" proclaims the basic goodness of our children, challenging the expectations we have for our kids and refocusing our attention on our primary job as mothers: to help them become exactly who they are.

"Mothers as Social Justice" investigates the link between motherhood and changing our world for the better, citing the subtle ways in which mothers are already social justice warriors as well as developing perspectives for when greater action is called for.

Finally, "The Fierce Mother Lineage" formally names the structure of an unbroken bloodline bending toward the already existent awakening as a result of the unique and universal experience of motherhood.

Throughout the book, I reference the "Lojong slogans," a set of fifty-nine short teachings by Atiśa, an Indian meditation master. I have always loved the Lojong slogans for their pithy relevance to everyday life. They are also referred to as "mind-training" because they were created for contemplation by meditation students primarily concerned with being of benefit to others. To be of benefit to others, one must have a tamed mind, so as not to project one's own agenda on to others. Not all fifty-nine made the cut for this book, not because they couldn't all be viewed through the lens of motherhood but rather because of my own personal relationship to them as a mother.

Each of the passages is an invitation to stimulate and investigate your own thoughts and feelings about the topic in question. Each idea could yield a full treatise. Some may touch a nerve, while others may not reflect your lived experience. With a deep and abiding love for and trust in your judgment and self-awareness, and longing to be of benefit to yourself, your children, and your communities, I offer just enough to empower your own contemplation and action.

You may choose to read this book cover to cover, to open to a random page, or to seek out a topic that feels urgent. When I first imagined writing it, I envisioned something that could be kept in the bathroom so that mothers could steal a flash of contemplation during the odd moment of sitting down. However you choose to engage with the book, it is my wish that it provide a deeper appreciation of yourself and your fellow mommysattvas, greater perspective and compassion for ourselves as we traverse this path alone–together, and the ability to see clearly (not always but often, and perhaps more over time) what is truly arising moment by moment and what is needed. I hope the book helps us all feel a little less alone. I also hope that it might allow us to recognize one another on the playground, in the supermarket, at the school pickup. To share that knowing glance and offer unspoken compassion, respect, and love. To perhaps go beyond what is unsaid and forge alliances that strengthen a new view and practice of motherhood.

Please do not mistake my thoughts for expert testimony on motherhood or Buddhism. I will always consider myself a beginner—in meditation, writing, and even motherhood— because every time I get remotely close to understanding any of it, it changes on me. New ages and stages for my son and for me, constantly changing circumstances, plus I am the most awkward person I know and am far from having my shit together. Just the other day I confidently called another mom by the wrong name and then saw my son kick her son in the shin. With all my meditation-induced presence and grace, I panicked and high-tailed it out of there.

What I *can* offer you, however, is honesty and realness. When it comes down to it, that's what I need more of in my life. I suspect that you do too.

The interpretation of the *dharma* as it applies to motherhood is my own. Anything that has been misconstrued or misrepresented is my error alone and not a reflection of the perfect teachings. I acknowledge the inherent limitations of my solitary perspective as an educated, able-bodied, middle-aged, middle class, cis-gendered, straight white woman with an only child. During the pandemic, I also benefited from being self-employed while having the stability and support of a salaried partner and help from my parents and our beloved babysitter, Giovanna (who is really my son's second mother). I was also able to get pregnant without intervention and gave birth vaginally. These were my experiences and are the position from which I approach motherhood and write. When I share from my personal experience, I am not trying to exclude anyone but to be honest from my subject position.

As compulsive as I am about reading others' experiences and as aware as I am of many simultaneously conflicting viewpoints, I have blind spots. Lots of them. My many privileges obscure the possibility of true objectivity, much as I wish for it. Being a mother may be the only place where our identities intersect. If this is you, I hope you can still see some of yourself in these pages. Know that I am still doing my homework and keeping my receipts, and please accept my apologies if these words fall flat or, worse, compound feelings of disparity or despair. Better yet, get in touch and tell me about it.

MATRESCENCE

WHEN MY SON WAS ABOUT THREE MONTHS OLD, I resumed seeing clients with disordered eating at my nutrition therapy practice. My mother took the Long Island Railroad into New York City and fed my son breast milk from bottles I'd pumped and stored in the fridge. Meanwhile, I walked to the office and wrestled to maintain focus on the individual sitting in front of me. Leaving my son behind felt as though I'd forgotten something essential; something more important than keys or phone, it was like a missing body part. It felt very wrong.

One day, after seeing a few clients and pumping during the short breaks between them, I headed home. It was fall, crisp and clear. Third Avenue was uncharacteristically empty, and I jay-walked. Stepping off the westside curb, I was an entrepreneur and nutrition therapist, someone who reflected back to her clients what their experiences meant about their evolving relationship with food and body. By the time I'd reached the eastside curb, I'd transformed into a mother again. Something intangible changed as I crossed the street that raised the curtain between my professional and my personal identities. Suddenly, work felt very far away. My focus shifted back to the timing of feedings and naps, how to best engage his developing mind, and wondering if I was doing an okay job.

Mother, daughter, sister, friend, dietitian, author, teacher, student, business owner, neighbor, citizen: these are some of the identities I juggle on a daily basis. They define me and they also completely fail to capture who I am. Questions of identity come up periodically for all of us, but on the path of motherhood those same questions feel even more confusing, conflicting, and important to understand.

Even for women who feel that their entire identity has been subsumed by motherhood, the actual metamorphosis of a woman into a mother is the least acknowledged change that occurs when a new child comes into the world. Yet the transformation that has occurred is profound, layered, unnameable, and irreversible. For many of us, it begins long before the moment of birth, whether with conception or the decision to adopt. For others, it comes at a moment's notice, when suddenly called upon to foster or care for a child. Regardless of when it happens, the process is essentially invisible. Recognizing the importance of *becoming* a mother is really understanding that a new being is born alongside the child, as yet unknown to others and to herself.

To become a mother is so enormous, universal, and determining of your life experience that it is on par with race, class, gender, ability, and sexual orientation. It can be a source of identity, connection, and access, as well as discrimination and exclusion. The driving forces behind becoming a mother have shifted dramatically in recent decades. When the pill came out in the 1960s, having sex no longer implicitly meant having children. The normalization of different paths to motherhood has allowed us to write our own stories. What was once assumed for a woman now not only has become optional but directly tied to her ideas about what gives life meaning and might lead to self-actualization.

The word "matrescence" was coined by anthropologist Dana Raphael in the 1970s to acknowledge the neurobiological changes experienced by women as they become mothers. Matrescence was later popularized by Alexandra Sacks (psychiatrist and expert in postpartum emotions) and Aurélie Athan (clinical psychologist).

Aurélie Athan has described becoming a mother as:

> an experience of disorientation and reorientation…in multiple domains: physical (changes in body, hormonal fluctuations); psychological (e.g., identity, personality, defensive structure, self-esteem); social (e.g., re-evaluation of friendships, forgiveness of loved ones, gains in social status, or loss of professional status), and spiritual (e.g., existential questioning, re-commitment to faith, increased religious/spiritual practices).

She has also called it "a life transition marked by disequilibrium and adaptation along with an opportunity for greater psychological integration and self-awareness akin to post-traumatic growth."

Identifying becoming a mother as a trauma—even if it was a much-wished-for trauma—is especially telling. In her novel *The First Bad Man*, Miranda July's protagonist, an adoptive mom, muses:

> If you were wise enough to know that this life would consist mostly of letting go of things you wanted, then why not get good at the letting go, rather than the trying to have? These exotic revelations bubbled up involuntarily and I began to understand that the sleeplessness and vigilance and constant feedings were a form of brainwashing, a

process by which my old self was being molded, slowly but with a steady force, into a new shape: a mother. It hurt. I tried to be conscious while it happened, like watching my own surgery. I hoped to retain a tiny corner of the old me, just enough to warn other women with. But I knew this was unlikely; when the process was complete I wouldn't have anything left to complain with, it wouldn't hurt anymore, I wouldn't remember.

Disorientation and reorientation. Disequilibrium and adaptation. Coming undone in order to be put back together. However you became a mother, the process involves an inevitable unraveling and reorganization of the self.

I imagine the transition into motherhood was not always considered a trauma. In the times when we were surrounded by extended family, becoming a mother was a communal event. Wise women witnessed and supported us through pregnancy, birth, and child-rearing. We were not alone. Each new realization, every "first" was experienced with others. They acted as our sounding board, these women; they had heard and seen it all. They would have told us when it was time to sleep, time to feed, time to change, what the different cries likely meant, how we ourselves could come into knowing.

Now the communal aspect of matrescence no longer exists for most of us, which makes the experience lonely, filled with shame and doubt. This is where the trauma comes from. Groups like the Mommy Sangha attempt to fill the void by virtually conducting one another through the passages of childbirth, loss, transition, and growth. Collectively, we rediscover an ancient language to describe the changes, the simultaneous shrinking and expanding of our world. We put the words together and share them to mark the momentous crossing over into unknown territory.

MANY PATHS TO MOTHERHOOD

THERE ARE MANY PATHS TO BECOMING A MOTHER and many intersections to being a mother. All of these determine the unique essence of your matrescence.

Whether you became a mother through pregnancy, adoption, surrogacy, or by marriage. Whether becoming a mother was planned or unplanned. Wanted or ambivalent.

Whether you had difficulty conceiving and/or carrying a pregnancy to term.

Whether you are straight, queer, gay, bisexual, intersex, asexual, trans, single or coupled, abled or disabled, fat or thin, Black, white, Asian, Latinx, Indigenous.

Whether you live documented or undocumented in your country.

Whatever the ethnic, cultural, faith-based, or spiritual group you belong to.

Whether you have access to any help or social assistance.

Whether you were younger or older when you became a mom ("geriatric pregnancy," anyone?).

Whether you are a trauma survivor.

Whether you had complicated pregnancies, miscarriages, previous or subsequent abortions. Whether you have ever lost a child.

Whether you have one, two, or more children, their ages and stages, and how those relate to your own ages and stages.

Whether you had motherhood-related mental illnesses such as postpartum depression, anxiety, OCD, or psychosis.

Whether your child deals with any physical, emotional, or learning challenge.

Whether you are caring for your children and aging parents or other family members simultaneously.

Your specific identities and their intersections define the nuances you navigate in each and every aspect of motherhood, making your unique matrescence worthy of exploration.

One of my dearest friends was diagnosed with an "adjustment disorder" when she was raising her three-year-old daughter— often alone and in the wake of two miscarriages and a long and frustrating fertility process, while teaching a full course load, fighting for tenure, and running a home. For her, as for many of us, the painful obliteration of self that is a normal part of matrescence was pathologized, leaving her feeling confused, ashamed, and alone. How I wish someone had taken the time to tell her that this obliteration of self was normal. That the "adjustment" to motherhood is not a smooth or linear process and that we all break in one way or another. That some parts of us are annihilated while others are liberated. What if the diagnosis had been "matrescence" and the natural response to that diagnosis was a prescription for community and rest and help, with the underlying understanding that it wasn't *her* that was sick, it was the prevailing culture, unsupportive of mothers, new and old?

It can be elucidating to contemplate your own matrescence. What was your path to motherhood? What was/is your relationship with your own mother, and how did that influence you when you became a mother? How old are you and how did your own ages and stages align with those of your child or children? What is your intersectional identity, and how has this affected motherhood? What aspects of motherhood feel universal and shared with other mothers? What aspects of motherhood feel unique to you?

WHEN MATRESCENCE HIT ME

THREE WEEKS AFTER I GAVE BIRTH, my partner had to travel for work, leaving me alone with our son for the first time. That morning, before he left, I packed up the diaper bag, buckled my son into the stroller, and walked to Central Park where I found a spot beneath a giant oak tree to unfold our picnic blanket. There in the shade, I breastfed him, precariously eating a sandwich above his head and periodically flicking off the crumbs I dropped in his hair. The selfie I took that day—our first together—was at just the wrong angle to perfectly capture my underchin and his near lack of a neck due to congenital torticollis. In the photo, you can see on my face a mixture of accomplishment and anticipatory anxiety. It was as if I were practicing for the next three days.

We didn't linger in the park because I was anxious to meet my partner at a café near his workplace before he hopped in a cab and headed for the airport. We sat there awkwardly while he held our son, him not wanting to leave, me not wanting to be left. When my son and I returned to the empty apartment, I felt an acute lack of supervision, the absence of any credentials related to keeping a child alive by myself, and the nauseating realization of how the next few days stretched out before me.

I used to love it when my partner traveled and I had the apartment to myself. I took advantage of those times by ordering Chinese and watching *The Real Housewives of* someplace or other, spreading myself out in our queen bed and encasing my body in all the extra pillows.

That first night alone with my son, however, I felt shaky. It was like when I first passed the lifeguard test and prayed that no one started to drown on my watch. When the takeout delivery guy knocked on the door, I was keenly aware of our vulnerability alone in the apartment. Thoughts of *Oh my god, it's just me... Why isn't anyone watching what I'm doing?... How am I supposed to know how I'm doing?* kept bubbling up. In many ways it had been "just me" all along, but the presence of my partner had made me feel safe; there had been a buffer in case of our son displaying a fever or a poop anomaly or in case of me just needing a minute to myself. Alone, I found myself walking a tightrope without a net.

I slept tentatively that night, waking easily at every shift and coo from his bassinet. When I rose in the early hours to feed him, the bedroom felt cool and vacant. He nursed and then we both went back to sleep. The next morning I stood by the bassinet and took a video of him waking up—in part to send to my partner, in part to prove to myself that I had made it. Swaddled in his blanket, blinking open his eyes, my son had no idea that a radical change had just taken place for his mother. I had leaned headlong into the uncertainty of that first night alone and made it to the other side without major damage to anyone involved. Before that night, there was an aspect of being human that I just did not know I was capable of manifesting. It was fierce and brave and soft and kind. It was a brilliant mess, and I was up to the job, no matter how arduous or stressful it may be. I was now, beyond any doubt or denial, a Mother.

THE THREE MARKS OF EXISTENCE

MOTHERHOOD IS AN AMPLIFICATION of the experience of being human defined by "the Three Marks of Existence." The Three Marks are the Buddhist version of Life 101 that describes the nonnegotiables we face if we navigate the world in a human body. They are suffering, impermanence, and no self. It is worth viewing them through the lens of matrescence.

Suffering is a basic truth of the transformation to matrescence. It is painful to become something you were not before, to leave one shore behind and swim toward another without being able to see it. It can feel agonizing to let go of dreams, plans, goals, expectations, privacy, and the illusions of certainty and control over your own life.

Impermanence is, as ever, the one constant. We experience change when we move through the various ages and stages of our own lives and the lives of our children. We struggle to realize what is happening, and just as we begin to understand and acclimate, the ground shifts beneath our feet once again.

The truth of no self concerns the reality that who we were and who we are becoming is blurry and unclear; we are both defined by our various identities and not at all defined by them because they cannot begin to capture the vast expanse of our being. The concept of no self tells us that what we think of as a solid and separate self does not truly exist; there is no clear definition of or separation between "you" and "me," between "you" before and after becoming a mother.

In recognizing the Three Marks of Existence and continuing to take the next intuitive step, we arrive squarely in our actual lives, touching in with an understanding of matrescence if only briefly and sporadically as it continues to unfurl around us. The life stories we write of working with suffering, impermanence, and no self through matrescence give our lives meaning, not despite the pain and uncertainty we encounter but because of it.

THE MANTLE OF MOTHER

ASSUMING THE MANTLE OF MOTHER is one part of the unfolding of matrescence. Some of us take this on easily while others of us struggle, but the experience is never one-note. Soft-spoken osteopath and Mommy Sangha member Aurelie shares:

> Matrescence for me was pure joy. I was so happy and on a complete high for quite a while. I felt like I was made for being a mum and that I was going to explode with that love and joy. But I also felt (and still feel) like a child compared to other mums and especially to my own mum. Overall, my identity shifted as I felt like I finally belonged and was a real woman. But it also showed me all my struggles around power, boundaries, wanting to be liked, and my own struggles as a baby, as a kid. It showed me how limited I am and how vast I am at the same time.

For Aurelie, becoming a mother felt like a welcomed arrival.

Others struggle to see themselves as a mother. Stina, a straight-talking lawyer and Mommy Sangha member, shares:

> The shift for me was a slow one. I remember being three months in and still feeling like the word "mother" didn't quite fit me, like a pair of new shoes that were too wide and kept falling off. I think it wasn't until Annabelle started

talking that I felt the word "mama" was part of my identity. In many ways, becoming a mother was like starting a new job. For example, my first job out of law school, I had the title of lawyer, but the reality was I had no idea what I was doing. I had read all the books, passed all the tests, but had never actually done the job. It took about a year before I felt remotely competent. I think it was when the new class of summer associates started that it clicked for me: I was now a mentor who had experience. Motherhood was similar in the sense that I was stumbling my way through the first year feeling like an imposter who knew nothing, and it wasn't until about a year in that I felt like I had earned this title.

My own experience was similar to Stina's in that it was gradual, tentative, and full of questions. For many of us, there is a vacillation between two extremes—this is me, and this isn't me at all. We are constantly shifting back and forth—am I, or aren't I? Assuming the mantle of mother is not a before-and-after moment that can be pinpointed but a stepwise process, uncertain at best, and often only appreciated in retrospect.

Our route to motherhood and how we assume that mantle are important components of our matrescence. They often reveal our hidden assumptions about and expectations for what a mother really is, how we think we fit the mold or don't, but they also allow us to own the physical, emotional, and spiritual hurdles that define our unique experience so that they become the ground we walk on.

THE JOYS OF MOTHERHOOD

IMAGES AND MESSAGES around the "joys of motherhood" are some of the most archetypal we absorb in our society: the glorification of the baby bump on the covers of magazines, advertisements featuring new mothers gazing into the eyes of their peaceful babies, composed family photos that seem to capture candid moments of mutual appreciation, fun family outings that don't reflect the hours it took just to get out the damn door. Effortless sweetness and deep uncomplicated love. Unfortunately, this portrayal of motherhood is unrealistic, oversimplified, and dismissive of the holistic experience that is actual motherhood.

The truth about motherhood is that it is a total shitshow that involves every imaginable (and many unimaginable) experiences and emotions, many of which we are not going to like. If we react to our dislike of aspects of motherhood with shame and without giving ourselves the space and permission to simply feel the way we feel, we also remove the possibility of discovering any genuine joy or wonder. We have to open up to our pain, our dislike, our hatred even, in order to tell the truth about motherhood. It may be more than we bargained for.

If you are a mother who dislikes parts of motherhood, join the club. I often don't like playing with my child and I have exactly zero interest in homeschooling him. If you are a mother who dislikes most of motherhood, you are also not alone. Please find ways of supporting yourself, knowing that it will probably not be helpful to find someone or something that instructs you on how to "like" motherhood. Rather, find ways of allowing yourself to feel the way you feel, to move through that experience with curiosity and compassion, to permit yourself the authentically complex experience you need to have. In my experience, meditation has empowered me to feel the way I do, not the way I should.

THREE OBJECTS, THREE POISONS, THREE SEEDS OF VIRTUE

IF WE ARE EVER TO DISCOVER the unparalleled joy of motherhood, we must make room for our pain and suffering too. (By the way, meditation helps us do this; see page 73 for instruction.) As humans, we have a range of experiences, from the highest highs to the lowest lows. Our natural preference for pleasure over pain often causes us to focus our efforts and attention on making sure we have more positive experiences than negative. When we have positive experiences, we cling to them for dear life. When we have negative ones, we panic, try to sidestep them, and wish to transform them into positives.

A mind-training slogan I come back to again and again is "Three Objects, Three Poisons, Three Seeds of Virtue." The three objects are the things we like, the things we don't like, and the things we don't care about. The three poisons are grasping on to the things we like (passion), pushing away what we don't like (aggression), and numbing out to what we don't want to look at (ignorance). The three seeds of virtue are freedom from passion, freedom from aggression, and freedom from ignorance.

When you spend some time with this slogan, you begin to see how it is relevant to everything we encounter on a daily basis. As phenomena arise and events occur, it is with the three poisons that we manifest our first level of judgment: I like this, I don't like this, I don't care about this. A beautiful day at the park with a well-behaved child: like. Standing in the checkout line with a toddler on the verge of a tantrum: don't like. Another explosive outburst that might signal something deeper is going on: not ready to look at, ignore.

When we slow things down, however, we realize that there is a gap between the moment an event happens and that first level of judgment of like, don't like, don't care. In that gap, there is no judgment, only raw perception. Perhaps the body begins to respond in a way that gives rise to our judgment; perhaps there is something there we didn't notice before. We will always have a preference for pleasure over pain, but as we train with this slogan, we come to loosen our grip on how things "should be" and work with them *as they are.*

I will always choose a joyful moment over a painful one. However, by trying to avoid experiences we deem negative, we unwittingly rob ourselves of our real lives. We miss out on the richness of moving through the tenderness of difficulty, of trusting one another to navigate challenging moments, by which we might come out the other side prizing these opportunities to witness ourselves, to lean into the mess, to move toward one another. It is in cultivating a tolerance for and appreciation of our struggles that we can finally discover the joys of motherhood.

BABY BLUES

I WAS WARNED ABOUT WHAT COULD HAPPEN during the first few days after giving birth, that the rapid shift in hormones and neurotransmitters might cause disturbing, painful emotional fluctuations, which was out of keeping with what I had envisioned for the first few days of motherhood. I thought I was in the clear, until one night five days in, having woken up to feed my baby and feeling painfully alone in this endeavor, I lashed out, viperlike, at my partner. I can laugh about it now, but at the time that momentous departure from the bliss I'd expected made me question whether I was fit to be a mother.

The path of motherhood is filled with these tectonic shifts—sometimes abrupt, other times more gradual. The maintenance of an emotional steadiness—though understandably preferable as it would indicate and reflect our desire for a sense of control and ease of existence—would in fact be impossible considering the reality of those changes. Though all humans share a natural preference for ease and pleasure over pain and discomfort, it is our attachment to that alternate reality that in the end truly causes us suffering. When we practice regularly being with things as they are, even as the canyon opens up between wishes and reality, we can see ourselves.

Except when we cannot, and it is not surprising that in our most stressful moments, when resilience and cognitive flexibility are low, we may only become aware of ourselves after the fact. In these (and all) cases, patience and self-compassion are in order.

For many mothers, the baby blues are their first experience with the emotional upheaval of motherhood. Baby blues do not last; knowing the pain is temporary can permit us the courage to feel it, to release ourselves into it, holding nothing back. Paying attention to the specific texture of our experience may not feel good, but at least we will be in our actual lives, working with the moment-to-moment turmoil that comprises at least part of our path of motherhood.

POSTPARTUM OCD

IT HAPPENED FOR THE FIRST TIME about a week into my son's life. I sat in our nursing chair trying to arrange my healing episiotomy tear so it didn't produce searing, mind-numbing pain. As he ate, in my mind's eye I saw the repulsive image of myself dangling my son out of our seventh story window. The images came regularly for weeks: him rolling under the metal gates that lined the East River walk and tumbling into the water below, his body being slammed into a wall in our apartment—images of me harming this tiny, fully dependent being who I already loved more than I thought possible. The brutal awareness that I was physically capable of doing him bodily harm ripped through me. It is disturbing to even type these words, but I vowed to include them when I learned how common it is for the fears of new mothers to be visualized in this way.

Because I'm me and need to process distress openly, I spoke out about these ugly, gut-wrenching thoughts to my therapist and to my mom friends, despite the fear that they would think I was a psychopath or call Child Protective Services to have my son removed. What I learned was that postpartum obsessive-compulsive disorder (OCD) and the intrusive thoughts that characterize it are very common among new moms. Thoughts of sexually assaulting their child, drowning them in the bathtub, shaking a crying newborn. Upsetting enough as they are on their own, the attendant shame and terror of those experiencing such thoughts keep mothers from ever uttering a word, which only compounds their dread.

Postpartum OCD is generally a temporary psychiatric condition that may or may not be linked to chronic OCD and/or a history of trauma. Just as our internal organs must shift to return to some approximation of their original position, so, too, are our brain chemicals disrupted and trying to re-regulate. Postpartum OCD is likely a combination of that chemical reorganization coupled with the stark awareness that not only could harm find our child in a world that is at times cruel and chaotic but that it could also come at our own hands.

As the handy 12-step saying goes, "You're only as sick as your secrets." If you have ever had disturbing thoughts about harming your child, you are not alone and you are not broken. From a Buddhist perspective, the intrusive thoughts of OCD represent another example of how our thoughts are separate from us. We have passing thoughts of all varieties, including those that are distressing, yet they do not define us as humans or as mothers; they do not determine who we are at our core. Our thoughts also do not determine what actions we take. Our willingness to directly face the full spectrum of our complex and often confusing minds is the domain of the mommysattva.

POSTPARTUM MENTAL ILLNESS

WHEN WE CONSIDER HOW COMMON postpartum mental illness is—with 15 percent of mothers developing postpartum depression, 10 percent experiencing postpartum anxiety, and less than 1 percent (but still a significant number) developing postpartum psychosis—it is telling that this issue is not the subject of international attention and collaboration. Even less acknowledged is post-adoptive mental illness, as adoptive mothers face radical shifts in their lives that dramatically affect their physical and emotional well-being but are told, "Well, this is what you wanted."

Change is inevitable and often painful. When a woman becomes a mother, everything changes—her body, her biochemistry, her experience of the world, and how the world experiences her. It is natural and human for radical changes to rock our world. We tend to prefer our lives to feel somewhat steady, without dramatic plot twists; when these twists nevertheless come, it can take us some time to adjust both physically and emotionally. It is often during this tumultuous adjustment period that postpartum mental illness shows itself.

When I had to abruptly stop breastfeeding due to a spinal injury when my son was one, the changes in my physical and emotional health came too fast and furious for me to handle them in any organized way. Hormonal changes, chronic pain, altered sleep, and ineffectual support (I had a lot of support and it still was not enough at that time) caused some combination of postpartum depression, anxiety, and psychosis. It was a rocky year before I was able to find some sense of stability, and I continued to feel shaky for at least another year after that. To come through that period of change, I needed medication, therapy, meditation, help with childcare, and the unconditional love and support of my partner, family, and friends.

Once we realize things have changed in emergent ways during the postpartum or post-adoptive period, our job shifts to acknowledging these differences and accepting them. We begin the process of letting go of what was to make space for what is. Some of us find this process more difficult than others for a variety of reasons. Our meditation practice assists us in recognizing when circumstances have changed. Often this is only after the fact, and that is fine; once in a while we can recognize things as they change in real time or even recognize the warning signs of impending change and anticipate it.

Once we have come up to speed with what is—whether that be the physical or emotional changes of postpartum depression, anxiety, or psychosis—we have a choice before us. Do we accept this new reality and do what is needed to attend to it? Or do we remain in denial? It might seem easier—to us and for those around us—not to accept that we are in need of more support. Yet this would just be kicking the can down the road. Taking the courageous step of speaking our pain, asking for help, and hopefully receiving it is, in this case, exactly what the warrior mommysattva must do. If it benefits her, it benefits all of us. Everyone needs a model of self-compassion and radical self-care.

LOSING OURSELVES

SOME MOMS SEEM TO MAKE THE TRANSITION to motherhood seamlessly and painlessly. New-Zealander-living-in-Germany and Mommy Sangha member Emma shares, "I don't feel like my old self ever left me; it's just learning new things...having breaks from [my kids] is good, but I don't feel an aspect of myself is missing when I'm with them." For moms like Emma, matrescence feels like building on to who they were before, an addition to an already wonderful house.

Others feel significant parts of ourselves have been displaced— if not lost altogether, then significantly rearranged. This is how it has felt for me. So much of my pre-baby life was self-possessed. My partner and I have always been independent and nurtured our own individual interests in addition to those we shared. So my time, money, and efforts were basically all at my discretion. This contributed to an identity I adopted—entrepreneur, traveler, night owl, reader, drop-everything friend, art and movie and theatre enthusiast, Buddhist student and practitioner—and that defined how I moved through the world.

After my son was born, everything else took a back seat. My sleep schedule immediately shifted to that of an early bird. While I remained in the workforce, I intentionally crafted my schedule around his needs. I didn't read a book for the first three years of his life. Exercise and most movies and late nights vanished. Travel for pleasure abruptly stopped. Friendships, meditation practice, and Buddhist studies changed dramatically.

Of the Three Marks of Existence, no self (or egolessness) can be hard to understand to those of us in the Western world, where individualism is prized. But this Mark not only holds that there are no true separations between "me" and "you"; it also offers that there isn't really a solid and separate "me" and "you" at all. I love to geek out on this concept by reminding myself of how nearly all my cells (except for a few in a part of the eye) have been replaced several times since I was born, or thinking about how there are more bacterial cells on and inside my body than there are "me" cells. Who, then, is "me"? Who is driving this bus?

The identities we adopt cannot begin to define us. Are these things that we feel make up our identities truly the things that we value most of all? It is not that we should give up parts of ourselves when we become mothers, or at any other point in our lives, but perhaps we might hold on to them a little less desperately. When we concern ourselves with the collective good, the collective experience, the collective trajectory of the world, it is then that we wake up and realize our purpose and our basic goodness, then that our other identities can assume their rightful place in the hierarchy of where and how we direct our energy and compassion.

MOTHERING VERSUS BEING A MOTHER

CONSISTENT WITH OUR EMPHASIS on doing over being, mothering—the action—often receives greater attention than simply *being* a mother. The act of mothering contains within it elements of molding, shaping, guiding, with a focus on a desired outcome. Being a mother, on the other hand, is being who you are and allowing your child to be who they are. Mothering may easily venture into the territory of smothering, helicoptering, and editing our kids in real time—there's a sense of "doing it right." Being a mother involves inviting "beginner's mind," a Zen Buddhist concept that means approaching something with openness and a lack of preconceptions. Beginner's mind allows us to engage with our kids—and our own experience of motherhood—without a specific agenda, sharing present-moment space with them, and discovering each moment as it arises, levels off, and ultimately dissolves.

Every day we are likely to shift from one perspective to another: one moment we are being and the next we are doing, mother to mothering. In reality both are required, but perhaps just allowing ourselves to be a mother is needed slightly more—by our children, by ourselves, by other mothers, by the world. Our meditation practice helps us to recognize when we have shifted from one into the other so that we can assess what is actually happening, what is needed, and respond accordingly, skillfully.

FULFILLMENT

WHETHER YOU FEEL YOU WERE MADE for motherhood or wonder if you're worthy, you probably came into it with certain expectations. Our childhood experiences, our relationship with our own mothers, and the narratives about motherhood in the larger culture and our unique subcultures all contribute to what we think motherhood will "give" us.

Self-described expat mama, bonus mom, self-care coach, doula, and Mommy Sangha member Kelly describes motherhood as an "evolution into who I always was...the thing I was always looking for." To finally arrive at "the thing" we were always looking for is the dream. Many of us enter into motherhood anticipating something similar—a sense of having arrived, a feeling of finally getting it.

But the "it" is not the same for everyone. What true fulfillment means depends on who and when you ask. We all want our lives to be full and meaningful, but we generally have very different ideas about what that means. Is it about giving our lives purpose? Filling up something that was previously empty? Allowing us access to a whole different part of ourselves and the world?

Whatever our definition, one surefire way of discovering satisfaction and fulfillment in motherhood seems to be the capacity to remain aware of our expectations and yet to show up and be present for every part of our experience that actually materializes. The joys and the struggles, the confidence and the self-doubt. Sure, we will prefer the easy times, but in practicing being here we are liable to learn a thing or two from the difficult times as well. Motherhood is unlikely to play out as we anticipated, but what does happen, depending on our capacity to meet it, is likely to be much more fulfilling in the end.

TEACHER AND STUDENT

MOMMY SANGHA MEMBER EMILY (not her real name) was going through a bitter and messy divorce. She fled her controlling home in the middle of the night with her then three-and-a-half-year-old daughter and moved in with her parents. As her sixteen-year relationship disintegrated in front of her eyes, she walked the fine line of protecting herself and her daughter while trying to maintain some semblance of a father–child relationship for her child. The night Emily took her daughter to a socially distanced drive-through holiday lights display, she received the devastating news that her husband had filed false charges against her and was petitioning for full custody of their child.

The next morning, all Emily could do was sit on the couch and breathe as she tried to hold her world together. It was then that her daughter informed her that one of her stuffed puppies, previously known as Runs Up the Hill, was now to be called Let the Darkness Come. Emily shares, "My breath caught as I racked my brain trying to think where she could have heard that phrase before—in a show or a story?—but I came up blank. I cautiously asked her, 'Does Let the Darkness Come like the nighttime?' to which she replied, 'Oh no, he likes the daytime. But he doesn't mind the dark.'"

As her daughter matter-of-factly resumed her play, Emily contemplated how much she had to learn from her little Zen master. She writes:

> I realized that I like the daytime, the easy days, the happy memories. But how would my relationship with my suffering and deep pain transform if I could learn not to mind the dark? If I could breathe through the difficult moments

and embrace them, welcoming them and learning from them…Let the darkness come. Even though I am scared and weak and exhausted, let it come. Let me learn to live with it and love it as much as I love the morning light, which I know it will most surely bring.

When we become mothers, we become teacher and student. We teach our children, through our love and compassion, that they are inherently good and worthy. We show them that we are there for them no matter what, that we will always do right by them. We teach them discipline, how to treat others with dignity and respect, how to productively deal with conflict and communicate effectively, how to be affectionate, how to develop a nurturing relationship with their bodies, and how to approach life and a world that can at times be confusing, chaotic, and uncertain.

In turn, our children teach us to see anew, to have patience, to give up our selfishness, to let go of plans and expectations, and to rekindle beginner's mind. They also teach us, in simply being exactly who and how they are, how to approach our lives with openness, joy, and purity of emotion.

WORRY

I NEVER UNDERSTOOD why my mother worried so much. Why, on not hearing back from me immediately after a missed call in freshman year in college, she assumed that I had met with some horrible fate. What I have come to realize since having my son is that worry is a mother's love language.

We imagine all the scenarios that may befall our children. We project in our desire to protect, and in so doing we reveal our fears, vulnerabilities, and blind spots. Worry, by nature, stems from the difficulty to stay right here, right now. Our minds shoot forward into an imagined future to anticipate every permutation and combination that might happen. I find myself doing this in even minor interactions with my son. For example, when he asks for a drink of water, the situation ceases to be about ensuring he does so politely and starts to be a question of whether I'm raising a boy who expects women to meet his every need. I fail to stay in the moment and attend to what is truly happening because my worry carries my mind away. Thankfully, my meditation practice has trained me to recognize when I have gotten lost, to acknowledge that, release it, and return to the present moment, gently and precisely. Without that training, I could easily get lost in the worrysphere indefinitely.

Recognizing our worry and how it pulls us away from presence helps us to refocus our attention, to accept the pain of not knowing what the future holds, to trust that we have prepared our children to go forth into their own lives so that we can let go. They will get hurt at times, and that is a painful reality. But we are not doing them any favors by trying to prevent every little scrape and bruise, either physical or emotional.

SELF-DOUBT, OR *THAT* MOM

I'M *THAT* MOM. The one who didn't realize today was picture day. The one who runs in five minutes late to pickup. The one whose kid is a little "weird." The one who feels compelled to truthfully answer you when you ask, "How are you?" The one who doesn't quite fit in with the other moms.

What I reveal in these statements is how judgmental I am of myself (and that I enjoy an inordinate amount of privilege in that I don't have to worry about not being able to feed my child, for example). I am also well aware that those who are most judgmental of themselves are likely to be judgmental of one another. I'm working on this.

There is no shortage of polarizing issues for moms. The mom wars rage on regarding sleep training, vaccines, screen-time limits, when to buy kids a phone, how to approach vegetables and sugar, parenting styles, and discipline. Despite all the parenting books and philosophies, there is exactly no way to know who's right and who's wrong. We are all flying by the seats of our pants, and this can cause unknown suffering and self-doubt.

What we can do for ourselves and other moms is to acknowledge our suffering and to wish for its relief. A Tibetan practice called *tonglen*—also known as "sending and taking" or "exchanging self for other"—feels tailor-made for mothers. In tonglen practice, we courageously feel our own pain and the pain of others; we breathe it in, knowing that we can handle it. Breathing out, we offer cooling, soothing relief, peace, and ease.

When I am struggling with the self-doubt of motherhood, when I am feeling like *that* mom, I breathe it in. I willingly inhale the claustrophobic, shameful sense of not having figured out something that every other mom has. I breathe this in for myself and every mom who suffers this way. By breathing this in, I realize that we all suffer at times, that I am doing my best, and that my child is okay. Breathing out, I offer the wish for relief, for self-confidence, for trust in the path and practice of motherhood. Whenever we suffer in motherhood, we can breathe it in and breathe out the wish for the relief of our suffering and the suffering of all mothers who feel similar pains at one time or another.

Tonglen also gives us the chance to share our joys with others. When something wonderful happens in our mom lives, we breathe that in. Breathing out, we offer that joy and fulfillment to all moms, wishing for them an equivalent joy.

THE ILLUSION OF SEPARATENESS

WHEN THE 2020–2021 SCHOOL YEAR rolled around, the mom wars were in full swing. Depending on your geographic region's experience with the virus, your school's capacity for remote or in-person learning, your political leaning, and your own work schedule (not to mention your mental health status), you probably had strong opinions on whether it was safe and wise to send kids back to school.

It is our supposed differences that often define how we see motherhood: how many kids we have, how much money we have, whether we have additional childcare, whether our kids attend private or public school, our work situation, our political and religious beliefs, whether we live in a city or suburb or rural area. These things are just some of the qualifiers that seem to divide us. While it is true that our differences strongly influence our experience of motherhood, it is what we all experience that has the capacity to change the global perspective on motherhood.

Becoming a mother has the potential to cut through our differences and highlight instead what is shared. For Mommy Sangha member Emma, "Becoming a mum widened my perspective rather than narrowed it. I felt the beauty and sadness of being connected to other humans, strangers and all." For me, the sense of interconnection takes many forms. These days it's about how my son's exposure to his friends, YouTube, and the current political and social environment—all during a global pandemic—is influencing his language, his gestures, and where he places value. I am seeing how fluid and illusory the boundaries are between one person and another.

Vietnamese Zen master Thich Nhat Hanh has said, "We are here to awaken from the illusion of our separateness." Just as all beings wish for unconditional love, safety, and inclusion, mothers wish for the well-being of their children. A mother may believe that her child's safety and health is ensured by different means, but the core wish is identical. When we feel ourselves hardening into "me" versus "her," "us" versus "them," perhaps this is the time to recall Thich Nhat Hanh's words. To awaken from the illusion of separateness is our purpose as humans and especially as mothers.

MOM SHAME

FEW SITUATIONS FEEL WORSE than when my child is misbehaving, not listening, or being openly disrespectful in front of other people. Suddenly everything becomes black and white: other children are perfectly behaved, other moms have it all figured out, while my child and I are a mess.

In these moments I stop thinking clearly and shift into image-maintenance mode. How I respond becomes less about working with things as they are and more about performing what I believe is expected of me, of all mothers. Despite knowing how important it is to acknowledge my child's feelings, the actions I take are for the benefit of onlookers. I am desperate to resolve the issue quickly while appearing completely in control, which generally gives rise to the exact opposite: an amplification of my child's distressing behaviors and a deepening of my mom shame. If I could evaporate in those moments, I would.

I experience mom shame as regular shame multiplied by a thousand. When I forgot to send a family photo along with my child on his first day of kindergarten, the sensation I felt was that of a gaping hole opening up in my stomach and all my organs collapsing into that abyss. I immediately forgot the multitude of the other things I had done to prepare him for that day: all the thought and planning that had gone into making a COVID-era hybrid school model work with my business, all the documentation that had been submitted, the visit to the pediatrician for the annual checkup and vaccinations, how I had talked him through what was going to happen and how our schedule was going to be different every week. Mom shame obliterated all perspective.

Brené Brown, the University of Houston researcher of vulnerability and shame resilience, has said that shame needs three things to survive: secrecy, silence, and judgment. Because of the nature of motherhood and how we are all experiencing it individually and usually not in community, secrecy and silence can easily thrive. Judgment is a choice we make. Because of our desire to be better and because we live in this culture that tells us self-aggression is motivating, we are often harsh and judgmental of ourselves.

To work with mom shame, we need three things: the courage to unlock the vault where we keep our most feared secrets; to speak our experience—the full spectrum of our experience—out loud to trusted others; and to challenge the idea that self-aggression and self-judgment motivate us to be better. So we might develop self-compassion, give ourselves the benefit of the doubt, and offer ourselves some much-deserved grace, time after time.

MOM FRIENDS

FINDING OTHERS WITH A SHARED VIEW of motherhood is not easy. In the earliest days of motherhood, I was distressed to discover two seemingly distinct camps. There were the moms who when asked how everything was going would respond with a high-pitched and very suspicious "Great!" At the other extreme, there were the cranky, perspective-lacking moms who felt that everything was awful. Like so many times in my life, I continued to search for a middle way.

What I needed in a mom friend was someone who understood that the journey we were each on—alone–together—is filled with highs and lows, simultaneously challenging, humbling, satisfying, and heart-expanding beyond imagination. I needed friendships that left room for suffering and pain, knowing that feeling and expressing them did not in any way crowd out the deep love and gratitude we have for our children or our own individual experience of motherhood.

As if it's not hard enough to find mom friends, many mothers also experience shifts in their existing friendships. Depending on the various stages of life friends are in—if you are not all moms, if you are becoming moms at different times, if you are an older mom, if your child or you has different or greater needs than other kids or moms—you might find yourself dealing with rifts. For moms of older children, friendship changes can also occur once the kids move out of the home or get into new areas of interest that require intense time and focus.

I lost two significant friendships in the early years after becoming a mom. In both cases, these friends were not yet moms and didn't understand how my bandwidth and capacity for time spent on the phone or hanging out had changed. I could no longer drop everything to be there for them as I had done before. In both cases, these women went on to become a stepmother and an adoptive mother and, I imagine, to discover how matrescence changes everything.

Other friendships can withstand the transitions of becoming a mother. They are elastic enough to survive the moving-apart–coming-back-together nature of relationships during a period of enormous change. These friends are forgiving, steadfast, willing to feel and express their disappointment, to have patience with us. The shifting tides of our friendships in early and later motherhood are another aspect of the metamorphosis—beautiful, clarifying, and sometimes very painful—of matrescence. We do come out the other side, of course, but it's only after we have experienced some very real growing pains and learned what they needed to teach us.

THREE LITTLE WORDS

AS UNIVERSAL AS IS THE PATH of motherhood, there are so many variables and ways to experience it that many of us can't help but feel alone. Case in point: the coronavirus pandemic. While the experience of being impacted by the pandemic was worldwide, the age of our kids, their individual needs, our own work and financial situations, and our geographic regions all determined our unique experiences and the effects on our families.

When the 2020–2021 school year commenced, mothers were faced with an unsolvable dilemma: send kids back to school—sometimes for just one or two days a week—and devise an ever-changing backup plan that could accommodate each week, or keep them home and do full-time remote learning so that, even if it meant depriving your child of face-to-face contact with teachers and peers, there would be some consistency and ability to plan childcare with a minimum (though still extraordinary) level of maneuvering.

Once again, moms hesitated to share their thinking process and decisions for fear of judgment from other moms. And with good reason. Between the coronavirus pandemic becoming a vitriolic political issue and the hysteria around lost education and ruptured social–emotional development, tempers were high and opinions and judgments were flying.

Cat and Nat, the Canadian mom duo and authors of *Mom Truths*, captured the true underlying needs of moms in this moment in an Instagram post, providing a script for what to say in response to any mom's decision to send kids back to school, participate in a hybrid model, do full-time remote learning, or switch completely to homeschooling. The universal response was "Man, I'm so proud of you! I know that wasn't an easy decision to make." We will often need to hear three little words from our fellow moms, which can come in several combinations:

"I get that."
"I can relate."
"Yes, me too."
"Yep, same here."
"That's so hard."
"You're doing great."

Not to mention "I love you."

THE MYTH OF "ENJOY EVERY MOMENT"

I RECALL THE FIRST TIME I heard these words. I was waiting to cross the street after it had taken me the better part of an hour to get myself and my son out the door. My mind was filled with the new reality that mobility and autonomy were no longer mine. The moment my son finished nursing, the clock was ticking for me to accomplish whatever needed accomplishing before he would need to eat again; his diaper had to be changed before leaving, extras packed and planned for; potential changing spots mentally noted; I had to try to pee as many times as possible to avoid having to race back to the apartment.

An older woman arrived beside me, gazed down at my momentarily peaceful cherub, locked eyes with me and informed me, "It's gone in the blink of an eye. Enjoy every moment." I couldn't wait to get away from her. Clearly, she had some form of amnesia about the captivity and claustrophobia of these early days. Of course I was enjoying my child and the experience of motherhood, but I was also suffering—newly indoctrinated into the culture where moms are glorified in word but not in deed. My partner was at the lab, absorbed in his research, while I was trying not to wet my pants.

Mothers are scolded to enjoy every moment while everything spins out of control—their bodies, their time, their very sense of self. Enjoying every moment is impossible, of course, and aggressively oversimplified. The experience of motherhood is far too nuanced and complex to be reduced to this one emotional note.

No matter how fast it goes, no matter how we will miss the ages and stages once they pass, some moments of motherhood will feel utterly unbearable, ridiculously boring, enraging, or disheartening. Just as we teach our children that all feelings are welcome, we can give ourselves permission to feel what is actually arising in the full spectrum of motherhood. We can renounce the need to obliterate "negative" thoughts with toxic positivity. In fact, it is only when we allow ourselves to feel and go through difficulty that we finally discover the beauty of our full experience.

GOOD ENOUGH

WHEN MY SON WAS TWO, we started having conversations about how nothing is perfect. When he broke a part of a toy that otherwise worked fine, we discussed whether we could still love something that isn't perfect. Later, when one of his grandparents told him he had done something perfectly, he retorted, "Perfect is just an idea. Nothing is perfect."

British pediatrician and psychoanalyst D. W. Winnicott coined the phrase the "good-enough mother" in 1953. In his research, he found that children actually benefit from having a less-than-perfect mother. When our kids are youngest, we must respond to their every beck and call. This is how we help them form secure attachment. But that level of bodily and emotional attunement and availability that we have for our children in their infancy is not sustainable, nor should it be. As they grow, they become more and more capable, self-sufficient, and flexible. Failing them regularly and in tolerable ways is actually one of the essential ways we as mothers help prepare our children for a world that will be at times disappointing and frustrating.

For example, I have a note taped to the front door listing "snack, water, wipes" so that I remember these three essentials whenever we leave the apartment. Nevertheless, in the muddle of putting on socks and shoes, reminding my son to pee, and negotiating what outerwear to don, I sometimes forget to stock my mom bag. His disappointment when he asks for a snack and I have nothing to offer is difficult for me to tolerate, but there is value in him having to tolerate that difficulty as well. In these moments, I apologize and share his disappointment, and I also explain to him that I am concerned with many things before we leave so sometimes I forget something. He needs to understand that his mother is human.

By being good-enough mothers who don't make life perfect for our children, we are training them to tolerate discomfort, one of the most important skills anyone can learn. Not getting exactly what they want the moment they want it might not be their preference, but it may be what they need. They learn by experience that even though life (and their mother) does not always comply with their wishes, ultimately they will be fine.

The fruition of the efforts of a good-enough mother is a resilient child: a person who can ride the rollercoaster of life, appreciating the ups, tolerating and finding meaning in the downs, ultimately deriving value and richness from the whole experience.

Many of us will interpret "good enough" as "not enough" or "settling for less than the best." This brand of perfectionism is self-abuse of the highest order. Even if maternal perfection were possible, what would be the result? A fragile child incapable of living in the real world. There is a gendered aspect to this question as well: what does striving for perfection as a mother teach our daughters about how they should be? What does it teach our sons about the role of women and mothers?

We can recognize our own desire for perfection in motherhood as the wish to rewrite what went wrong in our own upbringing or a way to assuage the pain of our disappointments and unmet needs. Stepping into the role of good-enough mother can give our failures a sense of purpose and meaning. We can relate to them as teachers, as necessary lessons, not as admonishments and harbingers of doom.

THE PROBLEM WITH PRODUCTIVITY

DURING THE PANDEMIC, in our efforts to mitigate our anxiety or simply pass the time, many of us came up with projects to complete. Closet reorganization, wardrobe detox, deep cleaning. Some of us turned our bodies into the project, with the plan to re-emerge post-pandemic with a new physique. We wanted something to "show for" our time in isolation. Such pandemic projects highlighted our difficulty in just being and how we power over that discomfort by doing, doing, doing.

Mothers often struggle with the idea of "getting nothing done." After a day of meeting the immediate needs of our children—feeding, changing, holding, helping, soothing—we fail to produce a list of specific accomplishments and can therefore feel a lack of worthiness. God forbid a partner returns from a day of work outside the home to highlight the lack of clean laundry, the absence of a home-cooked meal, or the presence of a dust bunny or two rolling across the floor.

Our current paradigm of productivity equaling value fails mothers. It fails to recognize the power of their very presence—the fact that they continuously show up with attention and intention for their children—and how that presence influences the long-term trajectory of their children. It can drive mothers to seek out more and more to do in order to meet the culture's expectations for productivity, whether in the form of work, fitness goals, or becoming a domestic goddess. Eventually, something has to give. What amounts to productivity for the mommysattva seeking a sense of worthiness can start to crowd out her capacity to show up authentically for her children and herself. Who loses out here?

Instead of looking at those days when we "get nothing done" as falling short on productivity, view them as exceeding the average in terms of awareness, interest, and engagement. On the days we are tempted to label ourselves as nonproductive, perhaps we could instead reframe ourselves as exceptionally present.

A ROOM OF ONE'S OWN

IN BECOMING MOTHERS, many women give up a sizable portion of their personal and professional lives, only to find that they long for that other identity, creativity, something of their own. For some, motherhood is the deus ex machina offering respite from an unhappy or unfulfilling job. For others, it is the inception of a lifelong battle for work–life balance.

Eventually, many of us concede that something momentous has changed and that it is impossible not to be affected in the creative sphere. We are constantly split in terms of our attention and feelings of responsibility, desiring that sense of productivity, accomplishment, and personal satisfaction while longing to be with our children (and often suffering guilt when the latter is not the clear priority).

After the maternity leave, whether formal or informal, those of us who return to work or other endeavors often struggle with the expectation to resume business as usual, as if we can infinitely absorb additional physical and emotional responsibilities without our work being affected. I have often felt that I'm doing too much to do any single thing well, and I've wished several times to clone myself. Seeing my partner go off for the workday where he is privileged to have the time, space, and mental real estate for uninterrupted thought, I have often felt resentment.

The intensity of the early years demands we let go of some of that other life in order to fully concentrate efforts and attention on child-rearing. But when the cycles of closeness between us and our children grow longer, with them individuating and becoming more and more independent, the latter stages of matrescence find us desiring to reclaim something of our own—our work, a hobby, a creative outlet, or a corner of a room for our own.

We can acknowledge the loss, any anger or resentment we may harbor, the disorientation, the longing for what might have been, and remind ourselves that this is yet another stage of matrescence as we become the mother of an older child. Perhaps we might view this stage less as trying to recapture something from the past and more as discovering and integrating the different parts of ourselves, which must now include our particular experience of motherhood.

CONSTELLATIONS

THE WAY OUR PARTICULAR PATH of motherhood unfolds is influenced by countless intersecting factors—constellations, as I think of them. How old we are when we become mothers, our own cycles of self-awareness, our own balance of wellness and illness, where we are in our careers, whether we need to or have made peace with our own mothers, our upbringing, our demons. Our children have their own constellations—the ages and stages they move through, their specific physical, emotional, and spiritual needs, their differences, their temperaments, their ways of making sense of their world.

A mother's constellations intersect with those of her children. It is one thing to be a thirty-year-old mom with a teenager and something entirely different to be a forty-year-old mom with a threenager. Both are wonderful and challenging, but they are completely divergent paths because of the ways in which the constellations of mother and child—at countless moments in time—match up.

What's more is that a mother's and child's constellations intersect with the constellations of their environment, their culture, their epoch. Homeschooling a kindergartner while racial and social unrest escalate and a global pandemic rages during an election year is different to sending your kindergartner off to full-time school during otherwise relatively uneventful times (perhaps permitting a mother to finally contemplate her own needs with a little more space and time).

The ways in which our constellations align with those of our children, our environment, those of our partners, those of others around us form the basis of our particular story. They make our experience of motherhood unique, provide a context for why we struggle and thrive as we do, and always invite the practices of reflection and self-compassion. Becoming aware of those constellations provides perspective, helping us make sense of our experience, why we suffer, how we naturally respond, and how we might wish to course correct.

STRONG EMOTIONS

MOTHERHOOD IS A PARADE of strong emotions: joy, elation, awe, surprise, fear, grief, sadness, despair, anger, rage. We likely experienced all these and more at times before becoming a mother, but the ways in which motherhood cracks us open makes these strong emotions feel that much more searing and raw.

In our meditation practice, when strong emotions make it impossible to feel the breath, we have another option: we can turn our full attention toward the strong emotion. If anxiety, for example, is causing difficulty, we may turn our mind's attention to the sensations of anxiety—that buzzy feeling in our lips, the vibratory sense in our chest and belly. Without indulging the narrative we have about the emotion, we feel the sensations of the emotion, truly turning toward the feelings without holding anything back. Then when our attention strays and we do become absorbed in the "story" about the emotion, we gently escort our attention back to the sensations of that feeling.

Practicing with strong emotions in this way teaches us that there are no emotions that are inherently good or bad. Good and bad are judgments of what is innately neutral. On the cushion and off, when strong emotions visit us we can welcome them, scooch over on the couch, pat the space next to us, make room for them. They are nothing to be feared; they are both fleeting and impermanent and rich and deep in meaning.

BOREDOM

MUCH OF WHAT WE EXPERIENCE in motherhood can be described as boredom. We do many of the same things over and over again, day in and day out. During the pandemic, many people described this as perpetual Blursday, but mothers were already hip to the boredom of a concentrated, slowed-down experience.

Our culture is allergic to boredom. Step into any elevator or subway car and watch as people confront and then dodge the fact that, for a few minutes of their lives, nothing is happening. Out come the phones, the books. We suddenly need to pick at our nails. We have to do something.

From a Buddhist perspective, boredom is not a problem. In fact, it may be good news. It means that we are living our actual lives, not entertainment seeking, just being with things as they are, even when those things are not particularly exciting.

There are two kinds of boredom from this point of view: "hot boredom" and "cool boredom." Hot boredom consists of that initial itchy, twitchy response to the realization that nothing is happening. It's a restlessness that courses through the body, prodding the legs to run, the arms to reach for something, anything. It might cause us to pace, to raid the fridge, to doomscroll.

When we sit to meditate, hot boredom arises as the result of the contrast between the speed of our day-to-day lives and the slowness and stillness of our practice. I think of hot boredom as the breakers, the waves that crash over you, pushing you back toward the shore as you try to swim out to calmer waters. You have to move through this tumultuous phase to get to the stillness.

Once you get there, you have reached cool boredom. This is the place in which we make peace with ourselves as we are. We allow boredom to be as it is, to feel it, to stay with it. We see the reality that is our lives, right now.

In our meditation practice, cool boredom is where we begin to see ourselves honestly, adoringly, moment by moment. We are both feeler and observer. It is here that we notice our habits of mind, the ways in which we fill in every perceptible empty space with some form of drama or entertainment, and experiment with resisting that momentary urge without trying to modify the moment. When we practice staying with cool boredom, we truly slow down, stabilize, relax with life on life's terms. As numerous as the emotional extremes we experience in motherhood will be, most of our lives will occur somewhere in between, and that may be boring. This is not a problem; there is nothing to do about this except to notice it and be there without judgment.

LONELINESS

IF I AM LITERALLY NEVER ALONE, why do I feel so lonely? It's a paradox that mothers struggle with. The loneliness of motherhood is one of those things most people never speak of. The emphasis is of course on motherhood's joys, surprises, satisfaction, and delight. But running alongside all these experiences is often a troubling sense of being in this by yourself.

In the early days, the presence of our bodies equals our children's survival. Even as time advances and our bodies are needed less directly, they continue to be the home base for our kids. Days unfold with nary a moment to breathe alone between work, managing a home, and attending to meals, school, playdates, and other activities. We are often surrounded by friends and family, drawn near by this new person or persons we are raising, but the responsibility lies with us alone. Because of the trend away from children being cared for by extended families, even if you are in a room surrounded by your people your experience of being there as a mom is decidedly different. Only the mother is so acutely attuned to the shifting needs of her child. Only the mother is pendulating between whatever conversation is ongoing around her and continuously monitoring what is happening internally and externally for her kids.

Friendships often change in the wake of motherhood. We are not able to spend time with the people we love in quite the same way, and that can chip away at our feelings of connection. Priorities shift, and what motivated us to connect with others can feel less pressing. It is difficult to locate your "mom pack" given the philosophical mom wars, and even if we do find our people it is tricky to seal the deal with quality time.

The loneliness of motherhood need not be a problem, but we can allow ourselves to feel that pain. Loneliness is a truth of motherhood as well as in a larger sense: we are always alone, together. We are born alone, we die alone. During the awkward moment between birth and death, we encounter infinite opportunities for connection with others, yet our relationship with ourselves remains private, unknown to others and in many ways even to ourselves.

LOSING IT

I HAVE LAID AN AGGRESSIVE HAND on my child on three separate occasions. In sharing this I want you to know that you are not alone. If you are a mother who has never snapped in this way, I bow to you. I wish I could have stayed on that side of the line, but, unfortunately, I crossed it. Now it's up to me to work with that reality.

The first time, it was an instant after he kicked me in the face, half accidentally, half intentionally, during a freak-out. The second, it was at the beach where, in full view of my parents and other beachgoers, he kicked sand up in my face, for which I smacked his knee. The third was at the end of a yoga class when, whining about getting more iPad time, he stepped on my hair, dragging it on the floor. In all three cases, my reaction was automatic, immediate, and without time for reflection. In all three cases, we were both shocked and devastated.

It is unilaterally wrong to lay an aggressive hand on a child. How can we teach them to be gentle and nonviolent if we cannot contain our own aggression (and please know that we all have the capacity for aggression within us)? Rightness is not the issue here. The question is what we do when we have crossed that line.

At the most basic level, acting out with aggression is human. Mothers are human. You are human. Humans make mistakes. We do not have infinite capacity for patience and tolerance. We have limits. The belief that mothers must be endless wells of faultless benevolence derives from the patriarchal society that pigeonholes us, limits us, generates self-doubt and perfectionism. In contrast to the rare moments of losing it, the majority of our lives as mothers is spent accommodating, adjusting, softening. It would be unfair and untrue to characterize ourselves based on an infinitesimal and exceptional moment. Doing so might unwittingly drive us to have more such moments—a self-fulfilling prophecy fueled by our fears and self-judgment.

There is likely to be a constellation of factors contributing to an incident of losing it—lack of sleep, garden-variety stress, a mismatch between our child's true needs in that instant and our crisis management skills, the accumulation of unsolved parenting problems. Taking this action does not come out of nowhere, but it is likely to seem as if it did. It doesn't matter how much you meditate, you probably never saw it coming. Knowing this, we can begin to pay attention to the buildup of aggression-inducing circumstances and tend to our own distress before it is discharged inappropriately. In the absence of this foresight, however, we need a way to work with our minds and hearts after such an incident.

What I have come to believe is that these moments demonstrate an utter loss of perspective. Space and time freeze; all awareness is sucked out of the room. We forget ourselves and our basic goodness. There is no understanding of before, during, and after, no consciousness of intention and impact, cause and effect, appropriate consequences of their (and our own) actions. Like our children when they hit, kick, spit, or destroy, when we act out in this way we have run out of skills. It is an act of deep confusion.

These situations also reveal our deepest-seated feelings, beliefs, and fears about motherhood and the dynamic between parent and child. We lash out when we feel the need for some kind of swift resolution—an immediate end to an unacceptable behavior, a "lesson" taught in a hot second. In these moments our aggression is the manifestation of our "mother dread"—that we are not in control, that we are not good moms, that our children have not learned to behave properly and might never learn. The act of laying a hand on our child represents how unimaginable it is to exist in a situation that is intensely uncomfortable. We respond to this overwhelming pain by slicing through it with a decisive action. We feel a momentary and intense need to cap it, contain it, control it. In reacting with aggression to abruptly end an unacceptable situation, painfully, we ensure an unacceptable situation.

Digging deeper and deeper beneath our aggression and our fear, we discover where we are most wounded. Indeed, these moments can be culminations of the trauma we experienced in our own lives, whether that trauma is with a capital T or a lowercase t. As the saying goes, "Hurt people hurt people." We don't cause harm unless we have been harmed. We are only capable of hurting others when we believe it is possible to rid ourselves of the hurt. Rather it is the capacity to hold our hurt, cradle it, embrace it that we see how we share this experience with all beings. Deepening our tolerance for our pain, our uncertainty, and our wounds is how we make a different decision when we arrive at those provocative moments.

SOCIAL MEDIA

FEW THINGS TRIGGER the compare-and-despair spiral more than viewing the highly curated mom life on social media. Letter boards captioning a "perfectly imperfect" quotidian scene, prescient quotes from young minds, odes to coffee and wine. The selective display in pictures and words of motherhood via social media has a particular way of creating unattainable goals for us as mothers. It can feel as if everyone else has figured out something we haven't—as if other moms can find something funny in the moment and not just in the retelling, as if they excel at the balancing act, as if there isn't a raw underbelly to their experience.

"Don't compare your cutting room floor with someone else's highlight reel" warns a useful maxim regarding the dangers of social media comparisons. It reminds us that social media posters are highly selective with what they share, while keeping the majority of their experience—including all the moments that spark shame, anxiety, and self-doubt—safely hidden. That we believe only certain aspects of our lives as mothers are worthy of sharing is discouraging. It reflects our near pathological obsession with control, happiness, and having it all together, and makes no room for reality.

Ninety-nine percent of the time, I choose not to share whatever snippet cut from the fabric of a day in the mom life might garner likes and laughs. At times I am exquisitely aware of what is unfolding—instances of confusion, fear, anger, or shame—and how it could be "spun" for social media. I have a deep desire to shatter the illusion of the quirky mom who simply rolls with the punches while maintaining perfect perspective, and to provide a window into the gritty, sometimes ugly, sometimes transcendent mom life. But usually the moment passes, and I am grateful for having noticed it, not for memorializing it in my reels.

WINE O'CLOCK

AS A SOBER MOM, I have strong feelings about the ways in which mothers bond over wine. It's not that I don't find it funny when a child refers to "Mommy's special juice" or when a mom homeschooling during the pandemic muses about her careful titration of coffee and wine. But having been there (though not while also a mom) I know that there is often a sordid flip side to the seemingly lighthearted and jovial relationship with alcohol.

In my memoir *Drinking to Distraction*, I shared some of the ways in which my drinking seemed to be enhancing my life but in fact was detracting from it. How I used alcohol to ease my social awkwardness but realized drinking altered my behavior in ways that aggravated it instead. How I drank to relax but realized that its effects on my body, sleep, and mood the following day were incredibly distressing. How I framed drinking as "me time" but how it actually caused me to miss out on those moments. When I became a mom, I was relieved that I'd already given up drinking because I knew that there would be situations in which I would wish to take the edge off, moments when I'd want to bolt, to not be there.

Moms all need ways of discharging the tensions that accumulate over the course of days, weeks, and months. We need a way of reassuring our nervous systems that they are safe, that there will be relief. Pop culture loves to encourage moms to drink—to connect with one another, to unwind, to be stylish and live her best life. But is wine o'clock a form of self-care? I'm not so sure.

I certainly don't think that everyone needs to stop drinking as I did. Most people would be capable of "mindful drinking" if they were willing to truly pay attention to their intentions and their own lived experience of drinking. Drinking provides such an "easy out" from discomfort that we must be very intentional when looking at our use of it. Mind you, this extends to "escapes" of every kind including shopping, social media scrolling, binge-watching Netflix, and emotional overeating. Our meditation and mindfulness practices help us stay with our experience long enough to recognize our deepest intentions, to discern whether the right next step is to lean into the discomfort or to anesthetize it.

WHAT OUR PARTNERS
DON'T UNDERSTAND (YET)

WHEN MY SON WAS THREE YEARS OLD and attending nearby daycare, I realized (though not for the first time) that my partner was missing out on something very important about parenting. Because of the location of his lab, it was his job to take our son to daycare. Each morning, after I wrestled my partner out of bed and tended to the many needs of our early-rising child, he put on his headphones, pressed Play on a podcast, and pushed the stroller out the door. Besides the safety concerns of distracted walking in New York City I was distressed at the thought of what he was missing out on by not engaging directly and inquisitively with our son on those daily walks. Having done the walk myself, I knew that my son was full of quirky observations and questions. What my partner didn't understand yet was that it is the most seemingly insignificant moments between our children and ourselves that can be the most precious.

The winning goals and graduations are wonderful, but they cannot replace our moments of transition, shared silence, noticing something together, or spontaneous conversation. It is the constellation of these tiny moments that gives our lives as parents richness and substance. This is why it is essential to pay attention, to give ourselves over to the moment, to look and listen and be curious. To sit down as teacher and sit up as student.

Perhaps in paying such close attention we miss out on some forms of entertainment, the ability to have a continuous thought, and the sense of knowing what to expect. But there is satisfaction in that sacrifice. It is not martyrdom but true generosity to show up for our children in a constant, interested, and receptive way. These are moments we will never get back; whether we "enjoy every moment" or not, the effort to show up for them is worth it.

In order to show up in this way, however, we must first surrender, fully and vulnerably, to the unknown. A mother begins this process of surrender while she is expecting, so that by the time a child arrives she has some practice. Her partner might need additional time to adjust. If her partner is male, he might have been socialized to not notice these small moments, to place emphasis elsewhere. But I don't believe this difference is hardwired.

As our son grew and became even more verbal and interactive, my partner did begin to understand the importance of paying attention, even during the in-between moments where most of life actually happens. It isn't something that he can articulate and he might not even be conscious of the change, but his attunement to our child has sharpened. At times, my partner needs me to witness him witnessing some small moment with our son. He gets my attention and then gestures to our child as if to say, "This is something important." As a result, his sense of satisfaction with parenthood seems to have deepened and become more nuanced, like he finally "gets" something that had previously eluded him.

SEX

SEX HAS NEVER BEEN EASY FOR ME. I was raised to feel that I had to defend my body against the desires of men, which confused the intensely sexual being I was inside and had learned to hide. Even within the safety of a committed, loving relationship, sex continued to feel dangerous, loaded with power dynamics, potentially humiliating. There were times when I felt I could relax, when sex became fun, a form of connection, release, and bliss, like when my son was conceived. But it has only been since he was born that I really feel I have stepped into who I am as a sexual being.

Right after giving birth, though, both emotionally and physically, sex was painful. I received a "husband stitch" when the attending obstetrician, a male (not my regular female OB), delivered my son and then sewed up my tear. The first six weeks during which my partner and I were told "No sex" passed way too fast for me as I struggled to accept the trauma my vagina had endured. I was ashamed of my continued bleeding, occasional incontinence, and, once we started trying to have sex again, my pain. My partner was exasperated and fearful, in having lost access to my body in this way and at the prospect of hurting me. I imagine he was thinking, *If we're having sex this seldom now, what will happen in five or ten years?* That first year or two was tense.

When a child arrives, a couple is changed irrevocably. Even as it can strengthen the connection, a new baby can destabilize parts of the relationship that we rely on—shared alone time, date nights, access to one another's bodies, sex. Especially in those early years, relationships are vulnerable, which can lead to resentment, contempt, accusation, hurt feelings, isolation, and disconnection. Sex can become transactional or withheld because we feel wronged, misunderstood, neglected, forgotten. Our changed bodies might not feel sex ready, whether the judgments come from our partners or ourselves. We might be tempted to exaggerate or downplay the importance of sex to sidestep our own fears and discomfort about understanding what has changed, how it's going, what it now means to us.

Before I could tolerate vaginal sex again, I found myself masturbating in a tentative way, in part because my body felt foreign and in part because I would sometimes pee myself when I came. Touching myself brought me back to my earliest discoveries of pleasure, the shocking realization that my body could respond to touch in this blissful way. When I think back on it, I realize I was reclaiming my body and my sexuality. It did not belong to my son, not my partner, not the OB who had remodeled my vagina. It belonged to me, and I needed to rekindle my relationship with that part of myself. The relationship I had with my body after the trauma of birth, and to this day, is one of reverence.

Over time—and in direct proportion to my partner's willingness to engage in the messiest and most monotonous parts of parenting—I have felt differently drawn to commune sexually.

Ironically, all the piss and shit and blood from my child's body and my own seem to have opened me up to the more visceral aspects of life. My cellulite bothers me less; I have gratitude for my droopy boobs and care less about how they move during sex. I am less self-conscious of my body's smells and sounds and textures. I can't say that I often feel sexy, but I do feel sexual, sensual, and I own that.

I continue to wrestle with the choice between sleep and sex. The former almost always wins out. But my mind is more open and attuned to myself in this way. I am more receptive to my partner, more in my body and less in my head.

AN EMOTIONAL ROLLERCOASTER

WHEN THE ORDER TO SHELTER in place of the 2020 pandemic first occurred, my general reserves of resiliency and flexibility were high. It was an inconvenience, sure, but my child was quite young and so the academic and experiential losses did not feel calamitous. I was comforted by the fact that he would not miss out on life-defining milestones like senior year in high school, graduation, prom, and likely not even have solid memories of this time. I was keenly aware of those losses in other families, as well as the much larger threats of illness, death, job loss, bankruptcy, small business closure, home foreclosure. That awareness was sobering and helped me maintain perspective for months. Despite the radical changes to our mobility and sense of safety, I could even appreciate moments of richness as the three of us cocooned at home, sharing one thousand square feet but often occupying the same one hundred square feet simultaneously. In the same heartbeat, I could experience gratitude, heartbreak, tenderness, grief, and rage.

Then George Floyd was murdered, in the wake of the murders of Ahmaud Arbery and Breonna Taylor and countless others. The Black Lives Matter movement swelled to an unprecedented degree, only to be dismissed and misconstrued as looting and riots. As the country geared up for a historic election, our incumbent fanned the flames of fear, rage, and neofascism. I read, in utter confusion and disbelief, the social media posts of people I attended high school with who claimed the coronavirus was a hoax that would magically disappear postelection, that I was a "sheep" to wear a mask, that "the best way to not get shot by police is to not commit crime." The accumulation of all these layers of injustice, violence, confusion, and ignorance chipped away at my resilience. I felt raw and frayed and angry. And very, very tired.

As "the summer that never was" drew to a close and we neared the start of "the school year that would not be," I lost whatever perspective remained. My meditation practice faltered, connections with my support network became more sporadic, my fuse grew shorter, and I couldn't shake feelings of dread about the months to come. Though the pandemic—like all things—would have a beginning, middle, and end, we could only guess as to what stage in proceedings we were at and when the end would arrive. Fumbling around in that uncertainty, many of us grew so disoriented that we didn't know if we were coming or going.

My emotional repertoire expanded to include despair, something I frankly felt unequipped to navigate. Up to that point I had experienced moments of despair—fleeting instants of doom and dread and loss of hope—but they were nothing like this deep, ever-expanding darkness. Words I had been using to describe my internal environment, like "stress" and "overwhelm," no longer captured the depth of my experience. I noted the desire to fast-forward through this period of time to brighter days when we could resume some sense of knowing what to expect from our lives, when the balance of our emotions would tilt toward the positive. Having identified the emotion of despair, I wished that I could repackage it somehow so that it would feel less threatening, all-encompassing, and god-awful. But I also recognized it as an opportunity to work with things as they are—the basis of the path and practice of meditation.

Motherhood touches every part of our lives, particularly our emotions and mental health. The coronavirus pandemic put all that under a microscope—the joys and the despair, the transformations and the entrenched neuroses.

SITTING IN THE SUCK

SITTING IN THE SUCK IS PAINFUL. Even if you are fully aware that it will pass, that everyone else is suffering too, the desire to escape can be overwhelming. This feeling is captured in the sentiment "Everyone needs more than anyone can give right now."

The Serenity Prayer asks, "Grant me the serenity to accept the things I cannot change, courage to change the things I can, and wisdom to know the difference." Sometimes changing the things you can control amounts to holding your mind and heart differently. Not doing anything in particular but trying to relate to how you are and how you feel differently. Knowing that the choice to sit in the suck—feeling it, breathing it in—is one of the few things you can control can shift that perspective.

WHO AM I NOW?

MOTHERHOOD CHANGES US IRREVERSIBLY. Our lives will never go back to how they were before our children. Matrescence isn't a single point in time but a long-term unfolding that continues from the moment motherhood begins until the moment of our death. The question "Who am I now?" will continue to arise as we move through all the new ages and stages of ourselves and our children.

Ten years from now, my son will be fifteen. He'll be thinking about college. Or not. He might have a girlfriend or a boyfriend. He might have ideas about what he wants to do with his life. I'm sure he'll have thoughts about what I did wrong. If I'm lucky, I'll be fifty-five, going on fifty-six. Perhaps I'll have more time to write. To read. To visit the friends scattered across the US and overseas. Maybe I'll be able to swim regularly again. Attend a meditation retreat. I'm hoping that there will be more continuous thoughts, uninterrupted by the moment-by-moment needs of others. I hope I'll want to have more sex. When I think about how my life is likely to change in the future, I can rest into the now. Show up. Appreciate the fleeting nature of this perfect moment.

Imagine your own life ten years from now. How will you spend the time you have reclaimed? What will you care about? Will you sleep in more? Read more? Travel more? What will you create? Where will sexuality and sensuality fit into your life? How will you reflect on yourself as a mother, woman, partner, friend, citizen?

However you are feeling right now, whatever you are struggling with, one thing is certain: it won't always be this way. Ten years from now—or twenty or thirty—you will still be a mother, but almost everything else will have changed.

MEDITATION

THE ENTIRETY OF THE BUDDHIST canon derives from a single simple practice: meditation.

The universe of mindfulness and all its principles, teachings, slogans, and practices emerged after the historical Buddha sat down for forty days beneath a tree and stayed with his mind's experience until he saw the nature of reality.

Before becoming Buddha, Siddhārtha Gautama was prince in what is now Nepal. He lived a life of luxury, protected from all suffering and presented with only pleasurable experiences. Without exposure to the outside world, he married and had a child. Then, curious about the outside world, he explored beyond the confines of his home and was immediately exposed to suffering for the first time. He saw a sick man, an old man, and a corpse. He was distressed to learn that sickness, old age, and death were unavoidable for all beings, and the experience roused in him a curiosity about the nature of suffering.

He also saw a monk and thought that living a similar lifestyle might provide the keys to understanding suffering. He left his wife, child, and home behind and set out to study with religious men. It is at this point in the story that every modern mommysattva says, "Hang on a minute. He did *what*?" With good reason. If the process of discovering we are awake is working with things as they are, then why on earth did he not stay in family life? Furthermore, from the view of karma, he was going to discover his enlightenment no matter what, so couldn't he have done that with the wife and kid in tow? If a mother discovers present-moment reality through the path of mothering, then surely the same is true for fathers? Yes. It is true. The story was written by men and handed down, generation after generation, steeped in patriarchal ideals that do not consider women and children. Nonetheless, on balance it worked out for Siddhārtha, so we Buddhists generally give him a pass for shirking his familial duties; however, it is still worth pausing for a moment to acknowledge the inherent contradictions in this part of the story.

The holy life did not give him what he wanted, so he turned to a life of extreme self-denial and discipline. His asceticism nearly killed him. He realized that neither extreme of luxury nor poverty would provide him with the answers he sought, and so he instead committed to something in between—the middle way. This is when he sat down, relaxed with his mind as it was, and began to see the truth about life: that suffering is inevitable, that our resistance to suffering only amplifies it, that there is a way to work with suffering, and that the path consists of meditation and its derivative thought, speech, and action.

Meditation is the foundational practice for the mommysattva—she who loves her child more than anything and wishes for them to have a good, satisfying life. Motherhood presents us with countless situations in which we might be attracted to one extreme or another—letting our kids run the show or clamping down with rigid control; becoming so enmeshed that our kids never establish their independence or turning a blind eye when they need our support; indulging every momentary feeling and desire or crushing undesirable emotions. These extremes reflect our natural human preference for pleasure over pain, control over chaos, certainty over uncertainty, but extremes of any kind are inherently in conflict with the realities of life and the wisdom of the middle way.

In becoming mothers, pleasure and pain are intensified. We buy our ticket, get on that rollercoaster, and hold on tight. How do we stay with our actual experience throughout the ride? Through the practice of meditation: by sitting with our experience, watching our habitual mind, inviting spaciousness by slowing down and allowing things to be as they are, and by coming back to the present moment again and again and staying. The practice of meditation forms the basis of how to relate to our lives. We may seek safety by indulging in pleasures or the seeming control of self-deprivation, but it is only in the middle that we truly experience our lives.

WHY WE MEDITATE

MOTHERS WHO MEDITATE are not putting on the rose-colored glasses. They are showing up for their actual lives. No filter. No curation. Just the pure, raw experience of the most powerful relationship in the world.

None of us begins to meditate because everything is awesome. We come to meditation with hopes and expectations. To be calmer. To manage stress. To lower blood pressure. To work with anxiety or depression.*

In some ways, meditation has become another thing on the mother's to-do list. In addition to everything else, she must carve out the time to sit and work with her mind, often with the expectation of preternatural calmness, benevolence, and unflappability. But this is not the point of it.

Mediation is not a problem-solver. It's not a goal-oriented practice. It isn't self-help or a means of self-improvement. It is much more subtle and important than all that.

When I finally committed to a meditation practice, I was newly in recovery and beginning a relationship. The hopes I brought to my meditation practice were to control my angst and agitation and to be the person I wanted to be with my partner. Twelve years later, I still suffer with my angst and agitation and I'm the same awkward person I have always been. But what I have gained from meditation is deeper than I ever could have imagined. Rather than erasing the aspects of myself I couldn't accept, I have opened to my full self. Even though I struggle and suffer, I can be with myself as I struggle and suffer. This capacity to show up with and for myself deepens my compassion for myself and others and helps me to show up for my son as he inevitably struggles and suffers.

My teacher Susan Piver says, "We don't meditate to be good at meditating. We meditate to be good at life." The point of practicing feeling the breath without manipulating the mind isn't to

Meditation is not appropriate for all people all the time. Meditation is meant to alleviate suffering but can intensify it for trauma sufferers. Always consult your mental health professional before beginning to meditate to be sure it's right for you right now.

become the preeminent feeler of the breath. Instead, meditation brings out presence, compassion, and daring in our lives and in the world.

WHAT IS MEDITATION, REALLY?

MEDITATION HAS BEEN defined as "substituting for your discursive mind another object of attention." The *what* of meditation can sound lofty: training the mind. But the *how* of meditation is insanely ordinary and, I would add, much more important.

In meditation practice, we sit and feel the sensation of the breath. The mind is permitted to be as it is while simultaneously being trained to have one-pointed attention. As I sit to meditate, for example, I feel the texture of my breath (sticky or smooth, shallow or deep). At the same time, I sense the breeze from the window brushing my upper arm and am conscious of my son in the other room—one of many thoughts that arise, level off, and eventually dissolve. I am not trying to get rid of them; the point of meditation is not to stop thinking, only to put them in their place for the time being.

I often think of meditation in terms of foreground and background. Feeling the sensation of breath is in the foreground of my attention. Everything else—thoughts, sensations within the body, as well as the sense perceptions of sights, sounds, smells, tastes, and other sensations outside the body—remains in the background. The border between foreground and background is never static; it moves constantly so that most of my overall attention is on the breath, now thoughts about what I'm going to make everyone for lunch, now the dull ache in my middle back, now the sensation of breath again. As long as even 1 percent of my attention is feeling the breath, I need take no further action—just be with it.

When that border between foreground and background dissolves and thoughts completely absorb my attention, crowding out present-moment sensation and awareness, I might get lost for moments or minutes at a time. And then something wakes me up: it is the mindfulness I cultivate by feeling the breath that gives rise to newfound awareness and allows me to see where I am in space and time, to acknowledge I got lost, and to have a moment of pure presence. *Here I am!* When I realize I am here, I can place my attention where I wish. And so I gently escort that attention back to the sensation of breath and begin again.

As mothers, we have countless moments like this. We are present with our children only to have a thought enter our minds that takes us elsewhere. We might ride that thought for a while until we realize we have gotten lost. Mindfulness and awareness bring us back—we see that we got swept away, we recognize the difference between the thought and being here now, we let the thought go, and once again find ourselves squarely in our lives.

This is the practice of meditation. Nothing fancy. No robes. No transcendence. Just relaxing with things as they are.

BEING VERSUS DOING

YOU MAY BE FAMILIAR with the adage that human beings might more accurately be described as human *doings*. Mothers in perpetual motion may need to hear this most of all. The most valuable part of motherhood isn't what we do but who we are and how we pay attention. Meditation practice is the training ground.

So many meditation techniques guide you to do something: to notice, observe, or visualize. As mothers and as humans, in my humble opinion, we need more emphasis on just being. The difference between doing and being is subtle. Guided meditations are a wonderful way to practice just being, or they can serve as a form of entertainment. Only you know if you are using it for one purpose or another.

I am not a scholar of the many different forms of meditation, so I cannot be truly objective. And I gladly admit bias toward one particular technique: *shamatha–vipashyana,* or mindfulness–awareness practice.

In this practice of peacefully abiding, we feel. That is all. It is deceptively simple but not easy. We feel the sensation of breath, and when we get distracted by thought we come back and start over. The breath—that involuntary reaction that keeps us alive, that we don't have to manipulate—is our home base, always there to welcome us back.

When we just breathe, we can just be. We can take a break from all the external and internal demands we (and others) place on ourselves. Slowing down, stilling the body, letting go of expectations, and not getting attached to thought create space inside and around us. We touch in with our own basic goodness and the basic goodness of our children, free from agenda and striving. We see clearly how we all deserve the benefit of the doubt and to be held in unconditional high regard.

Mindfulness of Body

THE FIRST ASPECT of shamatha–vipashyana practice is mindfulness of body. It can be tempting to rush over the establishment of the proper posture in order to get to that more seductive idea of working with the mind, but this would be a mistake. Without a body, there is no practice, there is no feeling, there is no awareness. Without a body, there is no mother. And mothers are particularly suited to (pardon the pun) embodying this wisdom. We truly know the outer limits of the body's capacity to hold and enfold life itself. If that's not *bodhisattva* activity, I don't know what is.

However, mothers often have a complicated relationship with their bodies. The damage done by the diet culture, the demands to "get the body back" after giving birth, the ceaseless feelings of "never enough" create a dynamic in which the body feels alien, problematic, like an enemy. Even just being exhausted from having a newborn, through birth or adoption, is enough to throw the whole thing off-kilter. Taking our seat in meditation practice is an opportunity to reclaim a respectful relationship with our bodies and to welcome ourselves back to ourselves.

The first of the Lojong slogans, "First, train in the preliminaries," reminds us to appreciate the preciousness of a human birth, that the rare fortune of being born into a human body allows us to relate to the *dharma* and have experiences that no other known organism is capable of.

I would add to this that the mother's body in particular is miraculous and should be regarded as such.

To establish your posture, take a comfortable seat, one that emphasizes the dignity inherent in stopping in the middle of this crazy world to work with your mind. The meditation posture is simultaneously relaxed and uplifted. If you are seated on a cushion on the floor, cross your legs loosely in front of you. If you are in a chair, sit so that your feet are flat on the floor.

Whether seated on a cushion or in a chair (both of which are equally spiritual, by the way), feel your body connect with the seat beneath you and give your weight over to it completely, rooting down through the sitz bones. Allow yourself to take up and fully occupy that space rather than trying to make yourself smaller in any way for any reason. Building from the ground up, allow your hips, spine, shoulders, and head to stack vertically. The pelvis should rest in a neutral position, neither pitched forward nor slumped backward. The back is strong, the spine is tall while respecting its natural curves, the back of the neck is elongated, and the crown of the head reaches gently up to the sky. The front body is open, soft, and receptive. You may allow your belly to relax and stop clenching it or holding it in. Allow the chest and heart to soften. Let your shoulder blades relax down your back and let the upper arms be parallel with the torso. Rest your hands, palms down, on the tops of your thighs. Play with their position so that they are neither pushing nor pulling your upper body. Try dropping them down by your sides, then bending at the elbows to create right angles and resting your hands wherever they land on your thighs. Let the hands relax.

Release the muscles of the face and the throat. The mouth is closed but not clamped shut, with the jaw relaxed, teeth slightly parted, and the tip of the tongue resting where the back of the top teeth meet the roof of the mouth. Allow the breath to be natural, in and out through the nose; no special technique is needed. Keep your eyes open, because this is a practice of wakefulness and being with whatever arises moment to moment, not a practice of relaxing or clearing away thoughts (which, anyhow, is not possible). The gaze is soft and cast down slightly at a point about six feet in front of you. Your eyes take in the full visual field without focusing on any one spot. You might experiment with imagining that your eyes are relaxing back in their sockets or that you are looking at a point in the middle distance.

This is mindfulness of body.

 ## Mindfulness of Breath

THE SECOND ASPECT of shamatha–vipashyana practice is mindfulness of breath. In this part of the technique, bring your attention to the sensual qualities of the breath: the feeling of air in the nostrils or brushing the back of the throat, the rise and fall of the chest or belly, the feeling of clothing moving against skin as you breathe. How each inhale happens without your needing to manage it. How at some imperceptible point the inhale turns into the exhale, and how there is a small pause at the end of the exhale before the body breathes in again, naturally. Rather than thinking about or observing your breath, you are feeling yourself breathing, feeling each unique inhale and feeling each unique exhale, in the present moment.

Never was I more cognizant of the breath than during the coronavirus pandemic. Suddenly, everyone was talking about oxygen saturation and ventilators as people with COVID-19 struggled to breathe. Then the national news broadcast the tragic murder of George Floyd and included some of his final words: "I can't breathe." Something many of us took for granted now occupied center stage. Many of us reawakened to the reality that breath equals life.

The breath—in meditation practice and in life—is our home base. As mothers, knowing we can always come back to the breath is a relief. It has always been there. It has sustained us our entire lives. It will be there for us until our final moment. Until then, the breath remains the thing we can always come back to.

This is mindfulness of breath.

Mindfulness of Mind

THE FINAL ASPECT of shamatha–vipashyana practice is mindfulness of mind. Here you place your mind's attention on the feeling of the breath as if riding waves. Maintain this connection with the sensation of breath even as you notice thoughts flickering like fireflies or passing like clouds. Just as the eyes continue to see and the ears continue to hear, the mind continues to make thoughts. This is not a problem or something you need to stop. There is no need to "clear the mind" while you meditate—this would be setting up constantly thinking mothers for inevitable failure. Instead, practice allowing your mind to be as it is while you choose to feel the breath. If you don't get attached to your thoughts, most of them will come and go on their own. They follow the predictable arc of arising, leveling off, and then ultimately dissolving.

There is no conflict between feeling the breath and allowing the mind to be; these two things can peacefully coexist. You might envision feeling the breath in the foreground of your awareness while your thoughts are free to do what they do in the background.

When one of those thoughts captures all your attention and you become completely absorbed, to the point that you have lost all connection with the feeling of the breath, know that this is also not a problem. Whenever you realize you've gotten lost, simply acknowledge the thought (you might say silently to yourself, "Thinking") and then let it go with a sense of precision, gently coming back to the feeling of the breath.

That moment of noticing you have become distracted is no reason to berate yourself or tell yourself you are a bad meditator; it is actually something to celebrate, because in that moment you are fully awake and have chosen to once again place your body and mind in the same place at the same time by coming back to the feeling of the breath. Noticing ourselves thinking *is* the practice, so it doesn't matter how many times your attention strays. Whenever you notice that it has happened, just gently walk your attention back to feeling the breath as the object of your meditation.

This is mindfulness of mind.

EYES OPEN

ONE CHARACTERISTIC OF shamatha–vipashyana that usually raises eyebrows is that the eyes remain open. Many of us have been exposed to the idea of meditation with eyes closed, as if the only way we can settle the mind and find some peace is if we shut out the visual world. I, too, came to the practice of meditation with this assumption and was momentarily disappointed when my teacher instructed me to keep my eyes open, with a soft, downcast gaze. But that disappointment was quickly replaced by a sense of wonder that I could in fact stabilize with eyes open.

There are numerous reasons as to why we keep our eyes open, ranging from the practical to the more philosophical. As moms, we are tired. If we close our eyes when we sit to meditate, there is a good chance that we will simply fall asleep. There's nothing wrong with that, per se, and at times a nap should take precedence over meditation. If we could learn to remain awake and alert while also relaxing with things as they are, however, we might discover a new part of ourselves and our experience.

Another practical reason for keeping the eyes open during meditation has to do with trauma. Many of us who have experienced trauma (whether with a big T or a little t) are prone to flashbacks, moments in which our bodies become confused as to whether something dangerous is happening in the present moment or whether it has in fact passed and we are currently safe. This may not be true for all trauma sufferers, but keeping the eyes open in meditation seems to have a grounding effect, anchoring practitioners to the present moment and always giving them the option to drop the technique if something starts to feel uncomfortable.

My favorite reason for keeping the eyes open in meditation is that we learn to discover peace and presence without ever leaving our environment. As mommysattvas, finding a perfectly silent and uninterrupted space and time for meditation is unlikely. When we learn to practice with eyes open, everything becomes practice. When we are formally sitting, we stay with ourselves and our experience, finding value in even a few intentional breaths. If we happen to have a longer uninterrupted practice, that's a happy accident—icing on the cake. Off the cushion and in our lives, because we have trained to find stability amidst the mess, we can more easily come back to the present moment again and again. The technique guides us to recognize when we've gotten lost—to see that we have become absorbed in a thought that is decidedly not in the present moment—and to come back gently and precisely to the sensation of the breath, the present-moment body, or the child staring up at us, needing our attention and openness.

MOUTH CLOSED

I GET TIRED OF THE SOUND of my own voice. Whether I'm repeating the same words over and over again, narrating the day as it unfolds, or simply engaging in the ongoing conversation with my loquacious child, my voice rarely has a chance to rest. A precious part of meditation practice for me is resting my voice or, as my teacher says, "relaxing the muscles of speech."

This is not self-silencing but an opportunity to have a contrasting experience. Resting the voice may actually allow us to find our voice. Sometimes it may show us that words are needless. If nothing else, resting the voice during meditation practice allows us to appreciate the silence, the rare moments when no words need to be spoken.

WORKING WITH THE MIND

LIKE SO MUCH THAT MOTHERS DO, meditation can feel like a form of "invisible labor." It may be tempting to dismiss sitting and breathing as doing nothing, yet such a simple practice is intensely active.

As we meditate, we are conscious of what is unfolding inside and around us. By stilling the body and training our attention on the feeling of the breath as it moves into and out of the body, we become awake, alert, and present in our actual lives.

Feeling the breath is what synchronizes mind and body, placing them in the same place at the same time. It sounds simple to place body and mind in the same place and time, except when you consider how often our minds are elsewhere. The body, on the other hand, is incapable of escaping the present moment. It is always right here, right now.

Not that we have any choice as mothers, but there is wisdom in staying with the body—in not being able to escape our lives when they are challenging, monotonous, unsatisfactory, or filled with self-doubt. Working with the mind teaches us to stay with and feel all the emotional states we might wish to evade.

The importance of mothers being able to not only know their own minds but to have a sense of unconditional friendliness for them in all their possible manifestations cannot be overstated. When we stay, we learn to work with things as they are. In working with my own mind, I have realized that I never really wanted to escape but rather to feel better equipped to tolerate, accept, and open to my life.

FEELING AND ALLOWING

APART FROM THE SPECIFIC instructions on how to establish mindfulness of body, breath, and mind, I have come to think of meditation as simply feeling and allowing. We feel the body as it is, the breath as it is, the mind as it is. And we allow them to be.

On the cushion, feeling and allowing means welcoming whatever sensations and states are present in the body—relaxation, elation, pain, tension, anxiety, fatigue. We don't have to like them to welcome them, but we can notice our preferences for some over others. Similarly, we permit the breath to be as it is, feeling how its sensations vary from moment to moment and practice to practice. Finally, we allow the mind to possess whatever texture it has in the moment—speedy or dreamy, slippery or steady. In feeling and allowing, staying with our lives as they are, we practice "holding our seats," quite literally being with things as they are.

Feeling and allowing on the cushion prepares us as mothers to be in a state of flow with our lives when we are not formally practicing meditation. To be intimately aware of what is unfolding inside and around us—the energy shifts, the fleeting discomforts, the rising of joy, the sinking of disappointment. Whatever is happening, we are here for it. We also sharpen our attunement to what is unfolding inside and around our kids, which helps us know what they are feeling, how they are responding in real time to those feelings, and how to help them hold their minds and hearts. Feeling and allowing, sensing and responding—these are like a call-and-response for life. We fine-tune our capacity to practice skillful means, often noticing that the most appropriate response is simply to notice, to witness, to be.

SLOWING DOWN

THERE IS A BLACK-AND-WHITE image in my mind, from my high school physics textbook, as I recall. A pistol fires and an apple explodes. To the real-time observer, the two events seem to occur simultaneously. But capturing the event on film and viewing sequential still shots reveals that it is a series of events that unfolds: the trigger is squeezed, the bullet is released from the chamber, the bullet travels through space, the bullet enters the apple, and the apple is blown apart. In my nutrition therapy practice, this analogy has become indispensable in describing how, although urges and habitual reactions seem to occur automatically, simultaneously, and instantaneously, there is in fact a sequence of events that, if we are able to slow down, we can observe.

One of the first off-the-cushion realizations I had after beginning to meditate was this capacity to see myself in real time, as if the camera to my inner observer had entered slo-mo while my consciousness remained sharp, giving me many more options in terms of how to respond. Many times, in the heat of the moment with my son, when I might otherwise lose it, I am able to see my temper rise, to quickly develop perspective on what is actually happening and what is needed, and to respond accordingly. Not always, mind you, but more and more with time and practice.

Meditation helps us to slow things down. What seem like instantaneous reactions—the angry explosion when our child breaks a precious object, the shutdown immediately following the rupture of plans—can be reframed as a sequence of events inviting skillful response rather than automatic reaction. We may realize in those moments that what is provoking a strong reaction isn't even the current moment but something that started hours ago—or decades ago—and respond accordingly. While we may not feel comfortable with these moments, they do offer us unique opportunities to see our habitual thoughts and actions clearly, to break harmful cycles, to soften rather than to harden against our children and against ourselves.

PRACTICE LETTING GO

WATCHING MY SON'S EYES CLOSE at the end of the day—
seeing him let go—always feels so tender and important. He
longs to be able to control when it is day and when it is night.
To speed up the nighttime so that he can start another day. Then
his body takes over; his eyes grow heavy, his breathing deepens,
and soon every muscle relaxes. All is well when he finally lets go
and rests into sleep. I think of these moments whenever I'm faced
with letting go.

As moms, we become masters of letting go. We let go of expectations, plans, previous ages and stages. This is why motherhood
is so clearly a genuine path to awakening. These are not easy realizations. Letting go is difficult. Part of why we cling so tightly to
our expectations is because we think they will keep us safe. But
days come to an end, things change constantly, eventually we will
die. It is in letting go that we are liberated to relax into reality.

In the simplest way, meditation helps us practice letting go. As
we sit and feel the sensation of the breath, we inevitably become
absorbed in one thought or another. We love our narratives, those
stories we tell ourselves, those fantasies that entertain and distract
us. Momentarily, they seem to protect us from the realities of
suffering, impermanence, and the interdependence of all beings.
But they are not real.

As we continue to practice, our preference for reality over
fantasy grows stronger. That preference strengthens our capacity
to recognize when we have become absorbed, when we have lost
the connection with the sensation of breath that anchors us in
the present moment. We acknowledge the thought, let it go—
releasing it into the ether—and come back to the breath again

and again. The more we practice letting go on the cushion, the clearer the choice to let go becomes off the cushion.

MEDITATION IS ORDINARY

SITTING AND FEELING THE BREATH is incredibly ordinary—boring and monotonous, even. This is not unlike much of what we do as mothers: speaking the same words over and over, repeating the same tasks day in and day out, sometimes not even being able to tell one day from another.

Our view of the ordinary, however, can significantly impact how we engage with it. Are ordinary tasks a chore or an opportunity? A burden or a chance to practice being right here in the now?

Meditation practice whets our appetite for realness, even if that realness is on the ordinary side. Our hearts grow wise by ceasing to constantly seek entertainment and exceptionalism and by being exactly where we are, working with reality as it is. It is in fact when meditation grows boring and ordinary that it presents us with the opportunities to really practice.

MEDITATION IS EXTRAORDINARY

CULTIVATING A REGULAR (if messy and imperfect) meditation practice creates a foundation of stability beneath everything we do. That is not to say that life becomes less of a rollercoaster, but perhaps how we experience the ride changes significantly.

From the solid foundation we create by holding our seats—feeling and allowing, staying with our lives as they are—we begin to notice the magic of everyday life. Training the mind to pay attention, to notice when we get lost, to let go of thought precisely, and to come back gently allows us to appreciate life's riches. The tiny moments that might otherwise go unnoticed. For me, it is the tiny moments that contribute to a sense of abundance and flow.

Meditation shifts our allegiance from fantasy to reality, and there is nothing more real than the present moment. Through meditation practice, we recognize our dwelling in the past as delusion, our daydreaming about the future as illusion, choosing to come back to the present moment over and over again.

MEDITATION AS SAND MANDALA

IN THE TIBETAN BUDDHIST TRADITION, monks take great care to craft beautiful, intricate sand mandalas, which they then ritualistically destroy. Our meditation practice is just like this.

When we sit to work with our minds, we acknowledge impermanence. The moment, the thought is here one moment and gone the next. But something enduring is also generated. In 12-step programs, this is often referred to as Step 0—the willingness to be willing. In sitting and engaging with each fleeting moment, we generate an intention, a foundational view, a way of being in our lives that allows us to show up fully for even the most repetitive tasks or difficult moments. We acknowledge that each moment is in fact new, potent, precious, and yet unexperienced.

While resting our mind's awareness on the sensation of breath, eventually something captures our attention and carries us away. It is the same as any other real-life moment in which one second we're right here, right now, and the next we have escaped into our minds. When we become absorbed in thought during meditation practice, we may stay there awhile but sooner or later something wakes us up. Something interrupts the momentum of whatever narrative we're caught in and reminds us, "Hey, aren't we supposed to be feeling the breath?"

This ability to wake up when we get lost is an indispensable skill for mothers. It can feel impossible to cut through and remember where we are in time and space when we are distracted by the speed of each day and the crush of everyone's needs. This is often when we find ourselves exploding or imploding and going down the mom-shame spiral. At some point between getting lost in thought and the implosion or explosion, something intercedes. We catch ourselves, seeing what is happening in real time, thereby offering ourselves some choices.

Meditation practice hones this capacity to catch ourselves, noticing when we get lost, strengthening the muscle needed to come back. The off-the-cushion impact of meditation practice is lightning-strike awareness, compassion, and wisdom—to see the implosion or explosion as it unfolds and to change course if possible, whether that means extending yourself some grace and compassion, putting yourself in time-out, apologizing to your kids, or simply feeling fully whatever emotion is coursing through your body and mind at that moment.

Even our external efforts are subject to the truth of impermanence. We cook meals only to have them eaten in three minutes or simply dumped in the trash. We clean only to have spaces dirtied again. We do the laundry only to have to do it again the next day. We work only to find our financial reserves depleted again. If, however, we can consider these ordinary, repetitive, mundane tasks in the same way we consider the beauty of sand mandalas, we can discover a fresh perspective and see each moment as it is. We can appreciate and give attentive and loving care to the creation and also the dissolution of these efforts.

IT'S NOT ABOUT THE SITTING

MUCH LIKE THIS BOOK, writings about the Buddhist view are all based on the foundational practice of meditation in which sitting—feeling, allowing, being with—is of paramount importance. Mothers are therefore faced with a choice: sit on the cushion, or do what is required for the care and feeding of our families, the living of our lives.

There is a significant patriarchal influence in the dharma, wherein the depth and duration of sitting practice are prized. But there is always a cost. If we were to devote ourselves to a life of practice, there would be no space for motherhood. If sitting were valued above all else, everyday life would be implicitly devalued. Even if the point of sitting were to show up in our lives differently, you can't quite have it both ways.

What if we don't have the time to sit? What if when faced with the rare discretionary moment, we need to lie down? What if on our way to the cushion, our child wakes up from their nap or cries out for help with their homework?

But what if instead of focusing on the ways in which we fail to meet the standards for practice created by nonmothers, we were to discover the infinite moments of our lives in which being a mother is the practice?

Mommy Sangha member Aurelie's answer to this question is to do what she calls meditating *with* the body:

I struggle a lot with creating a safe container and maintaining boundaries with my eldest, and she knows it, so she tests and pushes me constantly. I have learned to anchor boundaries in my body, for example, saying "No" from my body and not from my head. The moment she asks for more TV time and I say "No," she looks up at me with frustration, anger, or sadness to see if I will hold that boundary, to see if she can push further. When that moment comes, I feel the sensation in my body and I say "No" again but as if I'm anchoring my "No" in my bony pelvis. I feel the sensation of my "No" down there. It's a physical stance, and my kid feels it. She knows there is no more pushing.

The point of sitting to practice meditation is to be able to show up in our lives differently—openly, warmheartedly, compassionately. So what is "real" practice? If meditation is about feeling, allowing, and being with—doing what is required in any given moment—then are we not practicing all the time? This is why there is no part of motherhood that is not practice. There is no part of motherhood that is not the path to awakening.

IT IS ABOUT THE SITTING

EVEN IF THE POINT OF MEDITATION were how we show up in our lives off the cushion, doing the actual practice and living authentically are inextricably linked.

Something happens to us physically and emotionally when we still the body, feel the breath, and work with the mind. It is organic, cumulative, and a direct result of doing the practice. The changes that occur in the structure and function of our brains as the result of meditation cannot be acquired without the actual practice. There is no shortcut.

Meditation is the reminder and the analogy we need to guide our moment-to-moment existence. Here we are in the midst of our everyday lives. Our bodies are as they are. Our breath is always coming in and going back out. Our minds are constantly active, producing all manner of thought. Sometimes our bodies and minds are actually in the same place; often they are not. We see our stories about ourselves and our lives and how they are manufactured—often quite far from reality. We continually bring ourselves back, back, back to the moment, the one real, true thing: now.

Meditation practice doesn't have to happen perfectly or for long spans of time to have an impact on our real lives, our feelings, thoughts, and actions. Sure, it is wonderful to be able to set a timer and sit on a cushion. But it is equally good and valuable and supportive of presence when we feel our breath while sitting at a stoplight, as we wait for our child to emerge through the school doors, when we are feeding them. These moments of intentional attention matter. They gather merit, power our compassion, remind us what we are doing.

MEDITATIVE ACTIVITIES

MANY OF US ENGAGE IN ACTIVITIES other than meditation practice that also encourage the body and mind to be in the same place. Yoga, running, knitting, cooking, dancing—these activities can be done in a mindless way or in a way that prioritizes feeling, allowing, and being with what is, in the same way actual meditation practice does.

Motherhood offers us countless opportunities for meditative action. Feeding, changing diapers, playing, doing the laundry, bath and bedtime rituals can all be done mindfully. These meditative activities are the bridge between on-the-cushion and off-the-cushion practice. They are often where the awareness and insight gained from actual meditation practice are first evident. Noticing while nursing, for example, that you are conscious of each individual breath and the sensations in the body. Recognizing while putting your child to bed that you are feeling their sensations in your own body and that you are aware of subtle energy shifts the moment they occur.

Bringing the mind of meditation to other activities infuses them with a freshness otherwise not appreciated. It helps us make the link between what we are doing when we practice and how we experience ourselves, our children, and our environment.

MEDITATION, INTERRUPTED

FOR THE MOMMYSATTVA, distractions during meditation are just as likely to be external as they are to be internal. When we sit to meditate, we place our attention on an object—in this case the sensation of breath—and attempt to hold it there. But it's as if our kids know. As soon as our butt hits the cushion, they need a snack, help building a LEGO tower, an audience for their latest self-portrait.

Distraction is inevitable, even in a meditation session uninterrupted by external forces. Our attention is captured by sticky thoughts ranging from the most mundane—*What am I going to make for lunch…Must remember to buy toothpaste*—to the most important—*I hope she does okay on her math test...I can't believe he's getting ready to leave for college.*

Distractions should not be viewed as problems but rather as essential parts of the practice. It might feel good to sit down and hold our attention on the breath without distraction, but that would be less helpful to us in our lives off the cushion. It is the capacity to recognize when we have gotten lost and to come back—with gentleness—that is the heart and soul of this practice.

Whether the distractions are internal or external, one thing is true. Becoming distracted many times and having to keep coming back is not "bad practice," just as becoming distracted only seldomly does not automatically equate to "good practice." *Any time* you sit to work with your mind as it is—including recognizing and responding to distractions—is good practice.

MEDITATION IS FLEXIBLE

SOMETIMES OUR MISCONCEPTIONS about meditation keep us from meditating. One of the most common misconceptions is that meditation has to be perfectly consistent and of long duration to have benefit. If this were true, it would be very difficult for most mothers to have a practice at all. Fortunately, this isn't the case. Meditation can be messy, irregular, and spur of the moment and still be of great benefit, not just to the meditator but to everyone around her.

Meditation's flexibility is what makes having a practice possible for the mommysattva. It would be wonderful to sit at the same time each day, for ten or twenty minutes at a time, in the same designated place, and be uninterrupted. If you are able to do this, by all means do. Do it whenever you can. But if this is not your reality, or at least not regularly available to you, join the club.

Please don't let the practice you think you should have prevent you from having the practice you could actually manage. Letting go of the expectation for how meditation should be opens you to a practice that is fluid and flexible, one that changes as you and your life do. At one point in your life, this may mean practicing for a minute or two as you make that first cup of coffee, taking a few intentional breaths as you wait for your kids to finally put on their shoes, feeling the breath as you are cooking or waiting outside dance class. At another point, it may mean having a practice that is closer to your initial expectations of meditation. Give yourself permission to have the practice that works for your life and let that practice evolve, deepen, and expand over time.

BEGINNING

FOR ME, IT WAS SLIDING DOWN off my bed and on to the floor one afternoon while reading a book written by the woman who would become my meditation teacher. Before that day, I had read plenty about meditation but wasn't ready to sit my butt down and really do the practice. I don't know why *that* moment. Maybe the pain of being human just got to be too much, and I was finally willing to give in and admit that I wanted to do this thing called mindfulness–awareness training. I'm sure I thought it would change everything. And it did. It made me more thoughtful and aware. It didn't make me a better person, per se, but life is long. I'm doing my best.

I began to meditate about seven years before becoming a mom, so when my practice became less consistent, I had a longer-term practice to refer back to. Many of the moms who join the Open Heart Project Mommy Sangha, however, are brand-new to it. Either they have never meditated before or have dabbled but not established a consistent practice. The stability and consistency of a weekly half-hour gathering provides a container in which to practice together, no matter what we are holding—literally or figuratively. From that shared experience, many moms go on to connect with their practice in a conscious-if-not-traditional way—feeling their breath as they settle a child who has woken up in the middle of the night, becoming attuned to the sensations of dancing in the living room with a toddler, bringing their full attention to helping their youngster learn to ride a bike. These moments in which mind and body are synchronized begin to feed the formal relationship with a meditation practice, one that accumulates and reaches into every corner of a mom's life.

But it all comes back to that starting point. There is no magic formula. In order to begin, you have to just begin. Try it moments at a time, then minutes, then longer as your life allows.

HOLDING THE THREAD

MANY OF US BELIEVE that meditation needs to be unwavering and for long spans of time to matter, to be of benefit. Both personally and professionally, I've found this not to be the case. The research shows that as little as seven or eight minutes a day have measurable value. Personally, I've found that meditation is flexible enough to be nourishing and transformative even when very untraditional. The secret sauce for me has been to always maintain a connection with my practice no matter its formal manifestation at the time.

We can begin to establish a regular meditation practice by being realistic and gentle with ourselves. By holding our meditation practice with a light touch. Set an interim goal of five minutes three times a week for two weeks and then see how it goes. After two weeks are up, come back and reassess. If you were able to maintain that commitment, keep it up. If you crave longer sits, perhaps increase by five minutes or add days. If it was not possible to maintain your initial intention, readjust—for example, by sitting for two minutes upon waking or when your child goes off to school.

Designate a particular place for your meditation practice so that you don't have to choose where you are going to sit every time you decide to practice. At the same time, know that the place is not essential—all you need to practice is your body. Find a specific time of day that works, perhaps appending the practice to something you do regularly. For the first several years of my son's life, I came back to my cushion as soon as he fell asleep for his first nap. When he stopped napping, I had to come up with something else.

Over the lifetime of your practice, try to maintain some connection with why you do it. Read books about meditation practice and the *buddhadharma*, specifically those written by mothers for mothers. Join the Buddhist view with your other life views in a way that brings a freshness and new perspective to them. For example, I have incorporated a Buddhist view into my work as a nutrition therapist, into my relationship with my partner, and into finding ways to be more active in social justice movements.

Find ways of practicing with others, whether with the Mommy Sangha or a similar group, a virtual "accountability partner," or the community offerings on Insight Timer, for example. Most importantly, notice the quality of your life—how you hold your mind and heart—when your connection with your practice is strong. That lived experience is the most persuasive argument for continuing.

KNOWING WHEN TO LET GO

WHEN WE FIRST WENT INTO LOCKDOWN, I began a 108-day meditation practice via Instagram Live. I knew that I would struggle to maintain a connection with my practice and that others would too. Knowing that people expected me at nine each morning made it happen. After the last day, however, my practice fell into disarray. The school year had ended, a home-based summer was upon us, and there was no end to lockdown in sight. One of many things I lost at that moment was my meditation practice. I had to let it go.

Sometimes meditation just is not possible. The demands of each day swell to absorb every waking moment. Even if they don't, those rare moments of peace must be used for other more pressing self-care needs like naps and hiding in the bathroom. Meditation can also become just another thing on the to-do list we either check off or don't, something we should do rather than get to do.

This is a completely normal phase for the meditator, especially for meditating moms. It's wonderful if you are able to maintain a consistent practice, but given all the ages and stages we move through, particularly when our kids are very young, it may become necessary to let go of a formal sitting meditation practice for a while. The breath isn't going anywhere, and the practice has been there for thousands of years; both will be there for you when you are ready to return.

Like any long-term relationship, the one with our meditation practice moves through cycles. In committing to working with our minds for the long term, we don't have to fear temporarily letting go.

One thing I notice each time I let go of my practice is that every part of my life is already infused with it. I feel its presence: when I insist my child speak to me with kindness and respect and when I return the courtesy; when I steady myself at the kitchen counter and take a deep breath, feeling the weight of my commitment, of suffering, and of gratitude; when I let go of my attachment to a few minutes alone and welcome my child into my arms.

If and when you let your meditation practice go for a time, notice the quality of your life. Notice how you relate to the highest and lowest points and everything in between. Notice how your life has been influenced by the view and practice of meditation. This exercise is not meant to shame you into returning to a sitting practice; it is an opportunity to notice how even when you are not sitting, your practice is present.

COMING BACK

JUST AS THE BREATH PROVIDES the home base to which we can continually return, our meditation practice itself is always available to us. We may move away from it for days, weeks, months, or even years at a time, but it remains, awaiting our return.

Whenever I have felt the need to let my practice go, I feel its reverberation in my moment-to-moment experience for a while. It supports me and informs the subtleties of how I think, speak, and act. After a time, however, I often find an edge re-emerges. A certain harshness and lack of flexibility in my interactions with my son narrow my perspective and cause me to feel brittle, reactive, like I'm struggling to keep my head above water. This is when I know it is time for me to come back, gently and imperfectly.

The barriers to coming back to a meditation practice after you have let go are largely emotional—guilt for letting it go in the first place, doubt about the value of re-engaging with it, fear that we will only lose it again. It is human to feel these emotions; there is nothing wrong with them and in fact they represent our desire to be better. Accepting the mixed emotions we feel in coming back to a meditation practice softens us, helps us to lean into the groundlessness of uncertainty, acknowledge our fear, release our guilt.

What brings us back to a meditation practice is the evidence of its benefit in our lives, our underlying trust in the path, and the love we have for ourselves and others. Coming back should be gentle, a brief reintroduction practice, for example, rather than a grand gesture that only sets us up for failure in the near future. As we take our seats after a pause, we drop our resistance, let go of the past, and come back to the intention of being with ourselves as we are.

About three months after letting go of my meditation practice during the coronavirus summer—save for our weekly Mommy Sangha group practice—I had a morning where basically everything went wrong. The last straw was when my son's iPad crashed and I needed to give him my laptop, abandoning all hope of working during those prized moments of virtual school. At first I paced around the apartment in a fit of resistance, but then I encountered my meditation cushion and suddenly it became crystal clear what to do. I sat down and felt as if I had come home.

Coming back in my own time made me grateful for having trusted the path and process, knowing that I didn't have to force or trick myself into practicing when it just wasn't happening. In fact, to "just do it" no matter what would have been an insult to my practice. A vote of no confidence. Instead I let go, knowing that the relationship was strong enough to endure and to be rediscovered again and again.

MOTHERHOOD
IS THE PATH

IN 2013 I TOOK THE REFUGE VOW to become Buddhist. In this ceremony, one takes refuge in the three jewels: the Buddha, the *dharma*, and the *sangha*. I took refuge in the Buddha as an example of a human being—not a deity—who achieved enlightenment; in the dharma, or teachings of the Buddha, also translated as "the truth"; and in the sangha, the community of practitioners who are alone–together on the path to awakening. That was the year I began my nutrition therapy practice, what I thought would be my "baby" to nurture, love, and grow. In 2014 I got pregnant—almost exactly six months after my partner and I had decided not to have kids. And in July 2015 my son was born.

During my pregnancy, I stopped being able to absorb new information. I was participating in a Buddhist studies group in which we examined dense teachings. As my rapidly changing body had me switching between sitting on a hard metal chair and sitting cross-legged on the floor, I felt I had already left that circle of students and the academic experience of the teachings. I stopped attending when I was seven months pregnant—the sitting by then untenable—and in many ways put my Buddhist "studies" on hold.

Time slowed down. My body took charge and did not ask for input in the manufacture of bones and teeth. When I sat to meditate (often with my cat Rufus's body wrapped around my belly), I sensed intelligence in the individual coming to life inside me. Just as the instincts of my body had taken over, this person clearly possessed wisdom that was both separate and not separate from me.

In one way, my Buddhist studies ground to a halt when I became a mother. But in another—one I've come to regard as much more important—they had only begun. For many of us on a spiritual path, motherhood can feel like a detour. While devoted practitioners eschew daily minutiae to deepen their meditation practice, mothers stay behind to nourish, attend to, and lasso tiny (and then not-so-tiny) humans. It is tempting to place greater value on the duration and depth of a sitting meditation practice than on being in the trenches of feeding, bathing, soothing, and connecting with our children. But this would be missing the point of why we practice.

The power of presence has gained awareness in recent decades, due in no small part to the work of Jon Kabat-Zinn, who has banged the drum for this practice over the past four decades and created the gold standard of Western mindfulness in his mindfulness-based stress reduction curriculum. It is not surprising that in order to break into the mainstream, mindfulness had to be packaged in a scientifically validated standardized program (uncoincidentally designed by a white male). The masculine qualities that made it relevant to our culture are perfectly aligned with what we collectively value—rationality, eventemperedness, scientific evidence, righteousness. I love all these things, but they are only half the story. They fail to include the more feminine qualities of emotion, embodiment, and lightning-strike wisdom that culminate from the mind–body–heart connection. Fortunately, mindfulness itself is not beholden to our Western values. It is inherently whole—a healthy balance of masculine and feminine energies.

I managed to prepare for and take the *bodhisattva* vow in April 2016, when my son was nine months old. I'd considered taking this vow a couple of years earlier but could not connect with my authentic inspiration. At the time it felt like a sensible next step, but that was not good enough for the seriousness of the vow. Committing your life to be of benefit to others is not sensible. After becoming a mother, however, the call to formalize my role as a bodhisattva became more insistent. Motherhood made my world simultaneously bigger and much smaller. Though my attention was concentrated on the microscopic needs of my son, I also felt an intense urgency to create a world that is kind, compassionate, and sane for my child.

Traditionally, the great bodhisattvas have been male (as was the historical Buddha—yes, that same deadbeat dad who left his family and found himself or rather his no self). They are cited as inspirations because they form an unbroken line of individuals who have not "indulged in self-preservation." But in order to do the work of the bodhisattva, we do need to be preserved. If we are not to indulge in self-preservation, who then exactly is concerned with maintaining our survival, safety, and sanity? A monk may renounce his worldly possessions but rely on the shelter of the monastery and donations to his Buddha bowl. Who is filling up a mother's Buddha bowl? In many cases, the answer is no one. And so, the mother must walk that fine line of somehow preserving herself while also attending to the pressing needs of others.

A bodhisattva makes one central commitment: to put others first, holding nothing back for themselves. Who does this sound like? Putting others first is a way of being that comes naturally to mothers whose very bodies will suck the calcium out of their bones to build those of the developing child. Emphasis is also placed on the bodhisattva's quality of taking responsibility, something mothers are all too familiar with as they naturally slide (or are slid) into the role of default parent, default planner, default logistics manager. As mothers, we are constantly scanning the horizon for the needs of others, attending to the physical, emotional, and even spiritual ups and downs of our children one day after the next. This omniscient quality requires awareness that is both focused and expansive, not unlike that which we hone through meditation practice; we feel the breath and at the same time remain aware of sensations, sense perceptions, and passing thoughts as life goes on around us. This two-pronged awareness allows mothers to attend to the changing of diapers, to have the patience of nursing a baby destined to be a leisurely eater, to let go of plans and reading and mobility while also having a panoramic view of themselves in space and time and of how everything is interconnected.

Whether or not I had formalized my role as a bodhisattva, when I had my son I took that vow. We all do, no matter our route to motherhood. As a bodhisattva mother, every moment becomes "the path." Motherhood is the path.

WORKING WITH THINGS AS THEY ARE

WE COME TO THE PATH of motherhood with many, many expectations. We envision adorable, social-media-worthy scenes in our mind's eye and can't wait to enact them in real life. The problem is that real life feels no obligation to fulfill our wishes. Sure, we could mold our lives and our children and retrofit them to our desires, or we could accept them as they are and conduct ourselves accordingly.

The Three Marks of Existence—suffering, impermanence, and no self—perfectly conflict with the three basic human survival strategies. These are the preference for pleasure over pain, the desire to make stable that which is always changing, and the reductive tendency to oversimplify things to allow our minds to wrap around them—for example, thinking that "you" and "me" are separate and unconnected beings.

When we see how our natural tendencies predispose us to suffer, we can despair or we can vow to work with them. Working with things as they are means cutting through our desires and attempts to "edit" our lives in real time and instead engage with them with acceptance, a willingness to feel, an appreciation and respect for life's ordinary magic. The opposite of working with things as they are could be called "fighting with reality," like my son does when he has to pee but doesn't want to (and we all know how that turns out).

As far as it is from our natural desire to grasp on to pleasure and resist pain, there is enormous relief in working with things as they are. This is not resignation, which has the flavor of avoidance and disheartenment. Working with things as they are is courageous, engaged, and in the end much saner than the alternative. It's not always obvious or easy. This is why we train in being present—so that we can see clearly.

BEING WITH ATTACHMENT

IN THE MIDST OF THE CORONAVIRUS PANDEMIC, my son turned five. Due to the circumstances, our celebration was a much-diminished event: pizza and cupcakes outside in the garden with my parents and a neighbor. As sadness swelled in my chest, throat, and behind my eyes, I thought it was disappointment for him and his unsatisfying party (though he was more focused on the presents). But as I sat with those sensations, I realized there was something else: the day marked the end of his babyhood.

I have never longed to return to an earlier stage in his life or even truly felt nostalgia. I have enjoyed each and every age and stage (though not every moment) he has gone through in large part due to the capacity for authentic presence. I credit the practice of meditation for allowing me to actually be there for his first years. As time passes, however, I have felt the bittersweetness of grief; sharing in his excitement and pride as he grows up and grows into himself is coupled with letting the sweetness of each age and stage slip through my fingers.

Our inherent enlightenment is revealed through experiencing the impermanent nature of how phenomena arise, level off, and dissolve, by opening to and being with each fleeting moment as it passes. Few have as many opportunities as mothers do to notice what is actually going on. Each year, each day, each moment, we notice. We surrender schedules, naps, our expectations of ourselves, our expectations for our children, phases that were particularly sweet, "that little voice," kissing on the lips.

Noticing our attachments in motherhood is courageous and daring. The unfathomable love, joy, and bliss we feel during those moments of richness make us want to hold on tight. But hanging on would be fighting with reality. Showing up fully as these moments naturally dissolve gives us the opportunity to touch what is known as the "genuine heart of sadness," that deep, tender, boundless capacity we have for feeling and compassion.

When we accept what is dissolving, we are also liberated to show up for what is arising. The good, the bad, and everything in between. Whether it is the sympathetic joy felt in our child's first word or step, holding the space of her heartbreak, or quietly watching as he makes a difficult choice, being there fully for these poignant and important moments is the ground, path, and fruition of everyday enlightenment. This is how we elevate who we are and what we do as mothers to the level of spiritual practice.

ENLIGHTENMENT IS A MALE FANTASY

PLACING ALL OUR ATTENTION on the intellectual understanding of an enigma can be a distraction. There is absolutely nothing wrong with intellectual inquiry, but it can grow to be the entire point, especially for those of us educated to absorb material in a nonsomatic—even antisomatic—way. This style does many mothers a great disservice due in large part to the fact that time is limited and the mind must already track a thousand things at once. The way of enlightenment for all of us through the present, the sensorial, the embodied—mothers have little other choice. Which is very fortunate, actually. Your exhaustion and harried states might actually be working in your favor.

In Gesshin Claire Greenwood's excellent article "Enlightenment Is a Male Fantasy," she describes becoming so absorbed in the contemplation of a Zen koan about removing hulls from rice that she fails to remove the actual hulls from the rice she is sorting, so that everyone is crunching on them the next morning at breakfast. A different approach would have been to simply attend to the sorting of rice, directing her full attention—body and mind—to the task at hand. No big deal. No cookies. Just attention, on purpose. And isn't that a form of wisdom?

The structures and systems within Buddhism that fixate on the attainment of enlightenment are largely patriarchal. Much attention is paid to the monastic tradition of Buddhist meditation in which one leaves behind daily life to sit for days, months, years at a time. To commit to this path, individuals are required to eschew family life and the daily tasks required to care for it—something not usually equitably accessible to women.

Scientists have looked into what exactly happens in the brains of individuals who are able to practice meditation so frequently, deeply, uninterruptedly. As interesting as it is to understand what occurs in the brain when concentration is allowed to deepen, this information doesn't apply to most of us and least of all to mothers in nonstop motion internally and externally, constantly multitasking, coordinating, anticipating.

A "householder path," on the other hand, prizes the simple beauty of meditation in everyday life: how each seemingly monotonous task offers the opportunity to awaken to the nature of reality. What meditation can bring to that sort of existence is a one-pointed focus, so that even as we are rapidly switching between tasks, in each one we are fully there (at least some of the time). The emphasis in this view, however, is on the process. Not the endpoint of supposed enlightenment.

SECURE ATTACHMENT AND
NONATTACHMENT

IN AN EXPERIMENT CREATED BY developmental psychologist
Mary Ainsworth in the 1970s, known as the "Strange Situation,"
infants were observed exploring a new environment, responding
to the comings and goings of their caregiver, and reacting to a
stranger. Based on these observations, psychologists identified
their attachment style as secure, ambivalent, avoidant, or disor-
ganized. Secure attachment is the psychological gold standard in
modern parenting. When a child is securely attached, she understands she is safe and secure, that her needs will be met, that she
can confidently explore and thrive and individuate, that her care-
givers will be there when she needs them.

The language of attachment is also used in Buddhist philosophy, in which one of the greatest obstacles to enlightenment is
our inability to let go of plans, pleasures, and expectations—our
attachments. These are the things we think will lead to happiness
and safety but which waylay us in the end. Similar to the psychological language of attachment, freedom and growth come from
trust and letting go—parents letting go of a too-tight grip on
their children, children letting go of fears in order to explore their
world and know their own minds.

As mothers we practice nonattachment not by letting go of
our children to whom we will always be attached but by letting
go of our expectations of them, by letting go of our control over
situations, by letting go of a need for everything to be framed in
a positive light. Nonattachment for the mother seems to come
by finding a middle way of physical and emotional attachment
and allowing space to exist and expand over time between us
and our children. By trusting and letting go while remaining

present, we both ensure secure attachment and practice Buddhist nonattachment.

GIVING OURSELVES GRACE

WHEN A MOMMYSATTVA COMMITS to being of benefit to all beings, this includes herself. Each of us is also an other deserving of compassion, love, visibility, inclusion, justice, and joy. It can be tempting as mothers to sacrifice our own needs for rest, pleasure, and connection in favor of the needs of our children, partners, and others. But being of benefit actually means working with things as they are, noticing when our own needs must take precedence, and meeting those needs or asking for help. I hope that as we recognize the spiritual significance of the mommysattva more and more, we will feel empowered by one another to care for ourselves and to show up for one another when we need the extra support.

Mommy Sangha member Aurelie does a lot of "intentional resting" with her children:

I model rest, which is something that was never modeled for me. After the birth of my second baby, I had very little energy. I spent a lot of time with my two kids on my bed. We called it *câlins sur le lit* or cuddles on the bed. It's the most simple practice. And we all do it. But the intentionality is key because I didn't feel like I was "doing nothing." I was lying on my bed and I was being available for them physically, as if my body was a source of energy for them and I was letting them come and recharge themselves. We had a few books around, and I didn't need to be talking much or entertaining them much.

One of the many beneficial consequences of prioritizing our own needs is showing our children how we all share the same basic desires: safety, happiness, health, and ease. As a result, we also model for our children how women do not exist to accommodate until they break.

Like everyone, mothers deserve grace. From ourselves, from our kids, and from the world. Mothers were not created to be perfect, and perfectionism is self-aggression of the highest order. When mothers extend the same grace to themselves as they do to everyone else in their circle, life becomes more flexible, livable, sweet, and beautiful.

THE MOMMYSATTVA IS NOT A MARTYR

FOR MANY OF US IN THE WEST, the bodhisattva may resemble a Christian martyr; we are most familiar with the concept of someone who prioritizes beneficial acts toward others while simultaneously suffering the deprivation of care to herself. In reality, however, the world cannot afford the luxury of maternal martyrdom, and I personally have no interest in it.

The mommysattva must attend to her own needs as fiercely as she does to the needs of others. This obviously cannot be done in a vacuum. Rather than the mommysattva emptying herself into the world to be obliterated, she requires the individuals, institutions, and systems around her to fill her Buddha bowl so she can do the work she needs to do—the work the world needs her to do. If we all understood how interconnected we are, the need to care for mothers would become much more urgent, or as Pema Chödrön says, "We would practice as if our hair were on fire."

We begin this process by not holding ourselves or our fellow mothers to standards of martyrdom and perfection. By rescuing ourselves and one another from the cycles of mom shame and mom shaming. By calling out the mutual exclusivity of accepting ourselves as we are and always trying to be better, to do more, to self-improve and strive and achieve.

Recognizing its supreme importance—and removing the burden of martyrdom—elevates the path of motherhood to the sacred. When we ourselves acknowledge the sacred nature of every moment as mothers—and project that sacredness on to other mothers and the larger world as well—our lives feel less isolated, less claustrophobic, and more like an honor to be respected and approached with dignity. The work I do as a mother, meditator, and counselor is all in service of exploring and deepening my ability to acknowledge the sacred nature of being human. It's not easy but I cannot find any alternative.

ORDINARY SACREDNESS

THE BUDDHIST DEFINITION of certain words often has a much different feeling and tone than do the traditional Western definition of those same words. "Discipline," for example, is gentle and precise instead of harsh and militant. "Laziness" is an indication of disheartenment rather than a synonym for sloth. "Compassion" is sharp and wise, not always warm and fuzzy.

The same could be said for the word "sacredness." My Catholic upbringing would have me believe that in order for something to be sacred, it must be separate from the ordinary and transcend the tedium of daily life. But in the Buddhist sense it is how we engage with the tedium, indeed seeing it less as tedious and more simply as what is, that makes it sacred.

It's not as if the clouds part and the god light shines down on every word a mother utters, every little pair of newly laundered underpants she folds. And yet there is sacredness in every moment. We hold that sacredness with a light touch. This everyday sacredness is largely unfamiliar in our mainstream culture. It is the role of the mommysattva to cultivate an appreciation of the poignancy of everyday occurrences. To practice meditation in everyday life. To have compassion in everyday life. To embody wisdom in everyday life.

The ordinary is made extraordinary by the how. How we live our lives. How we hold our minds and hearts. The emphasis is placed on working with things as they are, instead of the common practice of wanting to be anywhere but here—wishing to somehow modify every moment, to make it less painful or more pleasurable. What arises is exactly as it should be, and how we engage with each moment therefore has the potential for transformation.

GIVING UP OUR PRIVACY

IN MY PAST LIFE, before becoming a mother, my alone time was plentiful. I erected defined boundaries around "me time" and defended it passionately; I could emerge from that time feeling fully recharged and was rarely at risk of not having access to alone time whenever I needed it. After becoming a mom, "me time" evaporated. Not even my sleep was unaccompanied.

This sudden and sustained lack of privacy beat me into submission. Difficult emotions like anger, resentment (mostly toward my partner), and longing flooded me for months, years. Ultimately, it broke me, and I conceded my long-held need for that separate time. I learned—and continue to learn—to relax into the lack of privacy.

"Welcome to the end of being alone inside your mind" begins the Brandi Carlile song "The Mother." In devoting our lives to the benefit of all beings, mommysattvas naturally give up their own privacy. Not only do we quickly lose the ability to shower or go to the bathroom without company, we also relinquish our ability to mentally shut out the world and crawl into our cocoons. We enter a protracted phase of constantly worrying about our children, imagining the consequences of our words and actions, considering the ways in which they will easily or awkwardly fit into the world.

Time and space alone are often severely lacking in the lives of mothers. Even in the rare moments of physical solitude, mentally and emotionally we've got company. Our children seldom leave our minds, and there is little respite from the worrying, replaying, coordinating, planning, and anticipating.

When we relax into the lack of privacy, knowing it won't always be this way, we might find we are satisfied with tiny pockets of time or space to be alone, to do what we want to do. If we need to, we can also become more intentional about how we find and defend those pockets of time and space in order to ensure that we have enough exertion left for those who need us. I think it's a little of both: softening into that temporary reality and protecting what we need to feel okay.

YOU CAN BE GRATEFUL
AND SUFFERING AT THE SAME TIME

THE LORE OF MOTHERHOOD is that it is a blessed experience filled with joy for which we should be unwaveringly grateful. The truth of motherhood is that we can be grateful and suffering at the same time.

When my son was approaching his first birthday, my life began to read like a sad country music song. My cat died suddenly; my friend tried to die by suicide; I ruptured a cervical disk, stopped breastfeeding abruptly so that I could take something (anything) for the pain, and had surgery on my spine; my dad had a stroke; my son broke his leg; and I developed a phobia to moths. What rhymes with "moths"?

Simultaneously, I was the happiest I have ever been in my life, marveling at a completely new side of my partner, in awe of the relationship building between my son and my parents, completely in love with my child, and seeing and experiencing so many things for the second time through his eyes.

What has been essential has been acknowledging both the gratitude and the suffering simultaneously. One does not cancel out the other. One is not more valuable than the other. Equanimity has been described as "the mind of no preference." Of course we will always prefer pleasure over pain, but knowing that, we can cultivate the mind of no preference in not holding on too tight to our joy or our agony while simultaneously acknowledging and appreciating both.

"AND" MOMENTS

"I HAD A VERY BAD DAY," my son will say sometimes when I finally convince him to get into bed at night. We could have had a wonderful, fun, interesting day, but whatever happened most recently stays with him, so if the bedtime routine became a battle, that is what seems to define his day. This is human, what is known as the "recency effect"—we are more likely to remember what happened last in a series of events and to accord that event more weight. At the same time, it is only part of the story.

As much as we practice acknowledging gratitude and suffering in the same moment, we may overlook these "and" moments, in which positives and negatives coexist. Our negativity bias—an evolutionary benefit that helped us learn from dangerous experiences so as not to repeat them—causes us to give more weight to the negative portion of our experience. If we struggle as adults to recognize this complexity, it is no wonder our children struggle.

When we fail to see the entirety of our experience, a rebalancing of perspective is in order. For example, my son and I began a bedtime gratitude practice in order to "zoom out" and get a more holistic view of the day. Recalling just a few of the positive things that we appreciate, in addition to—not to the exclusion of—what is considered negative, has changed his tendency to characterize the entire day based on bedtime battles. And mine.

THE FOUR IMMEASURABLES

LOVINGKINDNESS, COMPASSION, sympathetic joy, and equanimity—the four immeasurables—are said to exist in all beings in limitless quantity. Lovingkindness recognizes that there is no difference and no real separation between "you" and "me." Compassion allows us to feel another's pain in our own heart with a wish for its relief. With sympathetic joy, we share in the delight experienced by others. And equanimity provides the steadfastness and stability to ride the ups and downs of the rollercoaster of life.

The four immeasurables are not distinct entities; they are deeply intertwined and related to one another. When we see that we are no different from one another, we cannot help but feel another's pain. When we share in their pain, we also celebrate their joy. Lovingkindness, compassion, and sympathetic joy share a warm quality; they are the beating heart of our natural connection to one another. Equanimity, on the other hand, balances out the heat of the other three with its coolness.

The mommysattva sits right at the center of the four immeasurables, engaging them as the need arises, as if she were conducting a symphony.

LOVINGKINDNESS

LOVINGKINDNESS, OR METTA, is a wish for others' happiness. Seeing ourselves as no different from anyone else, we acknowledge that we all long for the same things. In the lovingkindness meditation, we say, "May you be safe. May you be happy. May you be healthy. May you live with ease." We offer these wishes to ourselves, a loved one, a neutral party, someone more difficult (an "enemy"), and then widen the circle until we include all beings.

Sometimes it will feel easier to rouse lovingkindness for our children, while other times it will feel more difficult. They might fit into the category of "loved one" at one moment and "enemy" the next. Connecting with the underlying meaning of loving-kindness—an unwavering feeling of goodwill—may help us stay steadfast in these wishes. Regardless of our momentary relation to another being, their longings remain unchanged and identical to our own.

Practicing true lovingkindness for our children as they grow up can feel less and less straightforward. We hold the knowledge of what we all wish for in our hearts, while at the same time we acknowledge that we might not know what form that must take for our children. We may wish them happiness and ease, but perhaps our definition of that conflicts with theirs. Allowing the wish for their happiness to rise above our need to be the solution and source of their happiness connects us with actual lovingkindness.

COMPASSION

DIFFERENT FROM EMPATHY, compassion is visceral and automatic. It is the heart that lurches when we hear that someone's mom is ill, that a friend has lost a pet, that our child was rejected by their friends. There is no thinking necessary with compassion; it connects directly to our most basic state of openness and love.

The Latin root of the word "compassion" is *pati*, which means "to suffer," and the prefix *com*, which means "with," so compassion literally means "to suffer with." Compassion has also been described as the ability to hold another's pain in our own hearts. Who on Earth does this better than mothers? Whether it stems from previously sharing a nervous system, straight-up biology, or our exquisite attunement to our children's shifts in energies, happiness, and suffering, a mother's capacity to hold her children's pain in her own heart knows no limits. It continues to expand beyond what she thought possible.

Compassion is the mommysattva's superpower. It is what allows her to see through layers of confusion to what exactly is arising every moment. To know what is needed and to rouse the exertion, vigor, and motivation to respond accordingly.

IDIOT COMPASSION

THE RELATIVELY RARE MENTION of mothers in traditional Buddhist teachings typically has to do with the practice of compassion. Either it's the throughout-the-ages-everyone-has-been-everyone-else's-mother bit or it's a reference to the archetypal compassion a faultless mother has for her child. But this limited view reduces both the mother and the practice of compassion to being one-trick ponies.

Compassion is much more than a warm heart. It is not always puppy dogs and rainbows. There can be an edge to it—a searing quality that cuts through the bullshit. The classic example of this is when a child is about to put her hand on a hot stove. Do you hem and haw "Sweetie, I don't think you should do that. You'll burn yourself"? No! You swat that hand away and explain afterwards. I'll take hurt feelings over a hurt body any day. Yet sometimes we practice the "idiot compassion" of not confronting the true harm and taking the path of least resistance.

Akin to enabling one who is addicted, idiot compassion subtly distracts us from working with things as they are. While true compassion requires that we move toward discomfort, idiot compassion lets us bypass the real work. Avoiding idiot compassion in our relationship with our children requires us to do our own work, to recognize our edges, to discern our "stuff" from theirs, and to become more comfortable with uncertainty and discomfort. Ultimately, taking this courageous leap toward the unknown becomes another expression of a mother's love—true love that isn't always nice.

SYMPATHETIC JOY

SYMPATHETIC JOY IS THE CAPACITY to feel another's joy in our own hearts. Just as compassion connects us to another's pain, with sympathetic joy we celebrate another's delight and pleasure.

In our relationships with other people, sympathetic joy can feel difficult. While the sharing of others' pain is visceral and automatic, sometimes the immediate experience of someone else's joy can be interrupted or deflected. Whether that stems from envy, a scarcity mentality, or some form of compare and despair is less important than simply noticing the difficulty.

Feeling our children's joy in our own hearts is less complicated. Their celebrations are our celebrations. Their delight is our delight. The purity and spontaneity of sympathetic joy experienced via our kids gives us access to the same heart quality with others as well.

EQUANIMITY

THE FOURTH IMMEASURABLE is equanimity, the cooling, balancing counterpoint to lovingkindness, compassion, and sympathetic joy. I think of equanimity as being the quality that allows us to ride the rollercoaster of emotion and experience, feeling everything with a modicum of stability so that life feels both rich and navigable. It is human to prefer pleasure over pain, but with equanimity we can see our preferences, work with them, permit ourselves our natural reactions while at the same time not becoming too attached.

Equanimity is not "it's all good" or "positive vibes only"; it is not a means of bypassing the raw and vulnerable realities of life without letting anything touch you. It is in fact letting everything touch you while simultaneously holding your seat, feeling and allowing, coming back to the present moment again and again.

Equanimity serves a particular purpose in how our children see themselves reflected in us. They are constantly searching us for reference points: *Am I normal? Do you still love me? This feels scary...help. I want to feel okay but don't know how.* Practicing equanimity telegraphs that whatever comes up for them, it is not out of bounds. Not that their words and actions don't destabilize us at times, but that they don't change the love we have for them, that they never become "too much" for us, that whatever arises becomes the ground for partnering to figure things out. Our equanimity provides our children with the confidence to plumb the extremes of their experience, knowing that we will always help them find a middle way.

THE SIX *PARAMITAS*

BODHISATTVAS, THOSE WHO DEVOTE their lives to being of benefit to others, make it their life's work to practice compassion. The basis for this compassion practice is the six *paramitas* or perfections. The six paramitas comprise generosity, discipline, patience, exertion, meditation, and *prajna* or clear-seeing wisdom. They are not separate from one another. The paramitas build upon and balance one another.

Generosity is warm. It helps us practice the nonattachment of allowing things (and people) to be as they are while giving of ourselves fully, not expecting anything in return.

Discipline is crisp. It brings a quality of joyful presence in which we discern what is happening and what is truly needed moment to moment.

Patience is gentle, permitting phenomena to unfold at their own pace, allowing our children to develop and grow exactly as they need to (and extending the same grace to ourselves).

Exertion brings energy and vigor to our lives. It introduces freshness and motivation to every day, even when we grow weary and bored.

Meditation is precise. It reinforces the practice of being here now, of synchronizing mind and body, and of doing one thing at a time with attention and intention.

Prajna cuts through to the heart of the matter by culminating the previous five paramitas. It guides us to emphasize one or another paramita, transcending confusion and seeing clearly. That piercing wisdom of prajna is softened by the warmth of generosity and so on, ad infinitum.

The six paramitas are whole as they are; they serve as a complete framework for the life's work of the mommysattva: the compassion master, the kind-hearted and discerningly wise one. From the microscopic to the macroscopic aspects of the mother's life and work, the six paramitas provide direction, inspiration, and the ground for deepening compassion.

GENEROSITY

THE FIRST OF THE SIX PARAMITAS is generosity: giving
without holding back, expecting nothing in return. Generosity is
symbolized by the mother's wish to give everything to her child.
The most important part of generosity is the intention driving
the giving.

Mothers are inherently thought of as generous, but it is
essential to understand the subtleties of authentic generosity.
According to the Venerable Thubten Chodron, generosity is
"dependent on the giver, the giving, the gift, and the recipient."
Generosity in this sense is inextricable from wisdom and compassion. Each act of generosity is spontaneously arising—not
repetitive acts of transmission but unique events influenced by
the constellations of factors surrounding them.

Genuine generosity is not about being a doormat, enacting *The Giving Tree*, or giving until you are empty. It is loving
unconditionally, unwaveringly, and openly, allowing others to be
authentically themselves, and erecting and defending boundaries
that protect ourselves as well as our children.

Generosity is letting go of attachments. It could be letting go
of strict screen-time limits during COVID, knowing when to drop
an argument with your partner, or releasing the desire to get your
point across. It could be letting go of plans, expectations of how a
day will unfold, specific hopes about who your child will become
or who you will be as a mother. Generosity can also take the form
of receiving: giving someone else the opportunity to give to us.

The opposite of generosity is stinginess, the fear that in giving,
something is lost. This comes from a scarcity mentality. I don't
know about you, but I have definitely caught myself being stingy
with my love and affection. When my feelings are hurt, when I

feel disrespected, when I don't know how else to communicate to my child that a behavior is not okay, I might default to this painful point. Only by acknowledging this, not by denying or pretending to rise above it, can I see my deeply human confusion and work with it. Owning the limits to my generosity allows me to practice true generosity.

Generosity connects us with our boundless capacity to love. It sharpens our priorities. By stripping away our delusions and our grasping after safety, generosity reveals the deep and indescribable love that we have for our children, for beauty, for life, and for ordinary magic.

ORDINARY GENEROSITY

THERE ARE THREE KINDS OF GENEROSITY. The first is ordinary generosity, the giving of comfort, material goods, and acts of service. Much of what we do as mothers is to practice this kind of generosity: feeding our children, clothing them, playing with them, and providing the comfort, normalization of their experiences, and compassion that is their birthright. Ordinary generosity may sometimes be giving others what they want, other times giving them what they need.

Everything we can hope to give to our children must begin with us. So much of the archetypal mother image is one of unidirectional giving. It is true that in giving unconditionally we also gain, but the mommysattva must also protect her own sanity. This is a form of ordinary generosity too: modeling for our sons and daughters that everyone deserves caretaking, time to restore, and physical comforts, and that a mother who cares for herself takes nothing away from her children.

A basic practice in cultivating generosity is to give an object from one hand to another. Something in the transaction gives us a bird's-eye view of the entire process: the intention and desire to be of benefit on one side and the vulnerability and openness to receive on the other. To benefit and to be benefited. We begin to see that there is no difference between giving to our other hand and giving to *another's* hand. Going beyond the superficial appearance of ordinary generosity we see true generosity, the kind that reifies the basic goodness, wholeness, and worthiness of mother and child and every being.

THE GIFT OF FEARLESSNESS

THE SECOND OF THE THREE KINDS of generosity is known as "fearlessness." Fearlessness—central to the mommysattva— is not the absence of fear but the willingness to work with it in an ongoing way, so that we stay engaged with our lives and the people around us.

I have never experienced so many fears as I have since becoming a mother. Early on, I joked that I wouldn't let my son eat hot dogs, grapes, or popcorn until he was twenty-five. I have fears about harm coming to him, fears about him being rejected by his peers, fears about the effects of climate change and political unrest.

At the core, these fears are about the inevitable suffering he will experience in his own life. Those fears make me want to shelter him, to not interact with others in ways that might become difficult or uncomfortable, to make his life as easy as possible, and to protect him from experiences that could challenge his fledgling self-image.

Facing my fears about my child experiencing pain allows me to transform them. By opening to life in all its manifestations, I am able to touch the truth: he will be hurt and disappointed by others; sometimes he won't be accepted; he'll struggle to see his own basic goodness at times; and he'll wrestle with his own natural human preference for comfort over the direct experience of discomfort. This is what it means to be human, and it is generous for us as mothers to allow our children to experience all of it.

Though his suffering will cause us both pain, the generosity of fearlessness guides me to release him fully into his own life with all its complexities, to remain by his side as he experiences the entire spectrum of his emotions, to teach him that pain is not to be feared but approached with openness and curiosity. Through our fear and pain we experience our authentic lives.

I cannot rid myself of fear, but I can vow to work with it directly and consistently: I can engage in the practice of fearlessness.

A mommysattva who works with her own fears teaches her children to do the same. Explicitly and implicitly, she helps her children learn not to be afraid of their own lives. How to have confidence and self-trust—in their bodies, in their emotions, in their special interests, in the ways in which they are different from others. Imagine a world consisting of individuals not afraid to be themselves, not afraid of working with their precise variety of suffering, not afraid to share their unique gifts.

SHARING THE DHARMA

THE THIRD OF THE THREE KINDS of generosity is called sharing the dharma—sharing the path of presence and how that is related to the Three Marks of Existence (suffering, impermanence, and no self). How I wish someone had helped me understand this when I was growing up.

Even before I formally "discovered" Buddhism in my thirties, I realized that learning to be comfortable with discomfort was likely the most important life skill I could ever hope to master. The fact that we suffer is not evidence of "doing it wrong," being negative, or not having gratitude. Suffering is a fact of life, unavoidable in many cases but not without meaning. It is how we encounter, engage, come through, and reflect on that suffering that makes our lives worth living and that gives us access to the richness that cannot be found in a life of only pleasure.

The truth of suffering has been the subject of many conversations with my son. We have discussed how all feelings are okay, even though not all behaviors are okay. I consider it a small victory when I hear him verbalize that he feels sad, left out, disappointed, lonely, frustrated, or angry. As painful as it is as a mother to hear her child in pain, I know that his capacity to feel pain is a strength rather than a weakness. The ability to stay with difficult emotions gives him the choice of how to respond to them. Together we have discovered countless lessons in impermanence. When toys break, even though he feels sadness and grief, he can also be overheard affirming, "Well, nothing lasts forever," and that he "can still love something even when it's not perfect." Experiencing suffering and impermanence firsthand gives him a window into the experience of others as well; he gets how painful it is to lose something you love, to be excluded, to feel embarrassed. He is beginning to understand no self through this empathy and compassion, through sharing, taking turns, asking himself how he would feel if someone treated him the way he's about to treat someone else, and intentionally noticing all the invisible ways in which all our lives intersect with one another.

The generosity of sharing the dharma with our children both builds a foundation on which they can grow and individuate and solidifies the truths of being human in our own lives.

THE GENEROSITY OF BECOMING A MOTHER

WHEN I WAS A TEENAGER and struggling to individuate from my parents, I hit upon the idea that when a couple is leaving the hospital with a newborn baby (at the time the only type of coming into motherhood I had the imagination to see), they should be required to sign a contract. In that contract, the parents would acknowledge the child is a separate entity and not an extension of themselves destined to fulfill their wishes, make their lives easy, or meet their expectations. It would be a sort of division of responsibility: the parents' responsibility is to provide shelter, support, unconditional love, and respectful discipline, gradually helping the child to become self-sufficient; the child's responsibility is to be him-, her-, or themself.

There is generosity in the decision to give birth, to adopt, to foster—to mother. That generosity can be muddled by the blurring of boundaries between mother and child—who they each are, what is expected, what is owed. Or it can remain pure, poignant, and sometimes painful in the inevitable separation that is meant to happen and that is in fact best for everyone. When we become mothers, we attach no strings, exact no debt. We have given a child life that is now theirs to do with as they choose. We can—and should—guide and support them, but we're not driving that bus.

DISCIPLINE

DISCIPLINE IS A COMPLICATED WORD for mothers. Many of us have our own difficult history of childhood discipline, so we seek to do the opposite, or at least something very different, with our own kids.

When I was a child, in part due to generational differences and in part to my father's own experience with parental discipline, deference and obedience were prized above autonomy and individualism. This caused much confusion about the overlap between discipline and sovereignty. I was encouraged to be who I was as long as it didn't challenge the control of my parents. My personality grew around that compliance. I learned to place greater value on garnering others' approval and bent myself to that will. The intention was love. The impact was control.

I'm attempting to walk a finer line, to do a subtler dance, and to notice the space between helping my child grow into a respectful, polite, responsible person and allowing him—encouraging him, imploring him—to become exactly who he is. It requires a different quality of attention, humility; it requires a willingness to fly by the seat of my pants rather than adhering to a rigid set of rules.

In the West, discipline is associated with consequences for violating rules. In parenting, discipline is usually meant to teach our children how to behave. The intention is to generate compliance, and in the absence of compliance there is punishment. This approach to discipline can often break a child or provoke strong rebellion but not necessarily teach them how to behave.

The origin of the word "discipline" is important to understand: discipline derives from "disciple" or "learner." This suggests the purpose of discipline is learning; it's a transmission of how to be a good human. When we implement discipline with our children, therefore, a useful question to ask is what are we helping them learn? Are we teaching them compliance and fear of consequences? Or are we teaching them cause and effect, self-sufficiency, empathy, and right action?

Discipline in the Buddhist sense is associated with the joy of being able to come back to the present moment again and again. It produces the capacity to see ourselves in space and time by encouraging the discernment of what is actually unfolding in that moment—for example, whether we are attempting to shape our child according to our (or the world's) needs or accompanying them on their path to maintaining wholeness. In this way, the precision of discipline tempers the ebullience of generosity, but it is not harsh. It is one-pointed, awake, and alert.

In our own lives, the discriminating awareness of discipline helps us find the balance between not too tight and not too loose. For example, we can enjoy the wine without relying on it to manage our stress. We can dress ourselves well and comfortably without regularly resorting to retail therapy. We can maintain structure and routine in the home while also knowing when to be spontaneous and flexible. In these ways, discipline finds connection with joy, richness, nowness.

PATIENCE

WAITING BY THE DOOR with your bag slung over your shoulder, asking your child to put on his socks and shoes for the fourteenth time. Leaning against the wall outside the bathroom while your newly independent little one takes care of business "all by herself." Resisting the temptation to get sucked into power struggles while staying the course of the middle way—dinnertime, homework time, bath time, bedtime.

Patience is like oxygen to a mother: we need enough so that we can withstand our children's testing of every limit but not so much that we get trampled on like so many doormats. Enough so that our kids have the freedom to pace themselves but not so much that our own schedules and needs are negated.

Patience is not the same thing as gritting our teeth or grinning and bearing it (though we are often quite good at that too). It is also not being preternaturally placid or calm. Patience is the antidote to boredom, aggression, restlessness, and unskillful anger; it is the willingness to work with whatever arises on our paths and to give ourselves, our children, and our surroundings the space and time necessary to respond.

Patience helps us with our tendency to lose it. When discomfort arises, we are able to note it as such, to open to it, to feel it, and to decide how to respond instead of reacting habitually in ways that might be harmful. We hone the willingness to be with things as they are, rather than to compulsively solve problems, check off the to-do list, wrap messy situations up in a neat little bow. Patience permits us to recognize how we might normally react in one way and choose to respond differently.

The opposite of patience is aggression and speediness. In practicing patience, we engage directly with our restlessness. We slow down our minds and bodies enough to allow situations to become spacious and clearer.

EXERTION

"THE DAYS ARE LONG, BUT THE YEARS ARE SHORT," goes a familiar line about motherhood. My partner often reminds me how at some point in the future we will miss these days even though they currently boast a fair amount of struggle and monotony. I'm sure that is true but, nevertheless, it can be challenging to maintain engagement, inspiration, and motivation in the day-to-day life of a mother. Yet this is exactly what is called for.

Exertion is the energy of giving a damn. Without a specific outcome in mind, exertion allows us to continually engage in our lives with freshness, connection, and attunement. Exertion is karmic, taking both a long view of our actions and their likely outcomes and a very immediate view of the importance of every moment. It is what allows us to see that our children need to run around outside despite our desire to collapse on the couch. It is how we temper our own volatility when our child melts down in dramatic fashion, seeing that what is actually needed is a cooling, balancing quality rather than a reactive, incendiary one. It is what helps us to show up enthusiastically when we are commanded "Mommy, watch this" for the sixty-seventh time. With exertion, we experience how our immediate and habitual desire to avoid suffering actually amplifies it.

When we are unable to rouse exertion, it is said to be due to laziness. Like so many words in our lexicon, however, laziness in the Buddhist sense takes on a less judgmental cast, especially when applied to motherhood. There are three kinds of laziness: ordinary laziness, becoming disheartened, and becoming too busy.

The first kind of laziness is called ordinary laziness. Sometimes we just can't rouse exertion and it's not really because of laziness at all. I have never met a lazy mom, so when this first kind of laziness seems to be at play, I believe something else is happening. Unmet personal needs for sleep, rest, connection, and inclusion; untreated mental illness such as depression or anxiety; and generally feeling unsafe due to the effects of trauma, racism, sexism, misogyny, or homophobia can appear as laziness. With this shared knowledge we are able to judge ourselves and one another less and show up and support more, which is the best use of our exertion anyway.

The second type of laziness—becoming disheartened—might appear to be a lack of exertion. In reality, this type of laziness is the product of impossible expectations set up by our culture and our overwhelmed response. When we can't seem to win in countless situations, our discouragement culminates in a a a why-bother sentiment. The antidote to disheartenment in motherhood is to reconnect with our values. What really matters to us? Is it living a picture-perfect life or the moment-to-moment presence that allows our children (and ourselves) to feel seen and heard, significant and loved?

The third kind of laziness is becoming too busy. It is not difficult to imagine how this form of laziness emerges in motherhood and how it could be mistaken for something else. In reality, it is our trying to do it all and be it all that prevents us from feeling as if we are doing anything well. This can also prevent us from engaging with a more expansive perspective with our kids, as we might like to. The antidote to becoming too busy is complicated. Many of us become too busy not because we want to but because we feel we have no choice. To say that becoming too busy could simply be remedied by reconnecting with our priorities and rejuggling them so that motherhood resumes its place at the top of the hierarchy is dismissive of what women and mothers everywhere are trying to do simply to survive. To counter the effects of becoming too busy, therefore, we must change the systems that require mothers to do and be all things at all times. This is a big ask and beyond the scope of this short contemplation. But it begins as an inside job, then extends to how we relate to other mothers, other women, and the world. In a more immediate sense, venting to and connecting with other moms helps.

MEDITATION

A SIMPLE DEFINITION OF MEDITATION is "substituting for our discursive mind another object of attention." In *shamatha-vipashyana*, or mindfulness–awareness practice, that object is the sensation of the breath coming into the body and dissolving out into the space around you. In this technique, the practitioner stills the body, settles the mind, and feels what is always happening—the body is breathing. The attention is not perfect or all-encompassing; we remain aware of our environment, both internal and external. We sense sounds and sights and other sensations and remain aware that the mind continues to think, all while training our attention on the sensation of the breath.

Meditation is the basis for everything we do as mothers—even if we do it imperfectly. It is the training ground and the analogy for being able to place our attention somewhere and hold it there, to recognize when we get lost, and to come back with gentleness and precision. It is the antidote to speediness, distraction, and overwhelm. It is the reminder to do one thing at a time.

Perhaps the most important thing that meditation teaches us as mommysattvas is to feel, allow, and be with whatever arises in our experience and to hold our seat, to remain present. We welcome all thoughts, feelings, and sensations, allowing ourselves to have our natural human responses to what we consider positive, negative, and neutral but not reacting habitually. Through meditation, we develop the expansive awareness that allows us to see ourselves in time and space, to see how we engage in repetitive thoughts and actions, and to make adjustments as necessary. We gain the steadfastness and equanimity to weather all storms and to stay with our experience, to open to it, modeling and supporting our children's capacity to do the same.

PRAJNA

PRAJNA, THE CULMINATION of the six paramitas, is clear-seeing wisdom. It possesses a searing quality that cuts through to the truth, what matters most in any given moment. When we see the truth—the illusory nature of safety, security, and certainty— we can relax with it.

Developing the wisdom of prajna is a continual process of shedding our defenses, our ways of not relating to reality, our ways of trying to have control, our ways of trying to sidestep our suffering. We connect with prajna by cultivating nonjudgmental curiosity and letting go of the need to know. As a result, we become more resilient, flexible, and fearless.

Our children pick up on this and come to see us as the ones who can provide the proper perspective in whatever situation. When they question their basic goodness, when they experience self-doubt, when they feel god-awful, the mommysattva who practices prajna can offer something no one else can: unconditional love, gentleness, and the reassurance that even though everything is not okay, everything is okay.

We know our children better than anyone. We know what they are really seeking; we know the ways in which they want to feel capable, how they want to make a difference, how they wish to contribute in meaningful ways, how they want to feel powerful. Prajna helps us help our children feel independent and in control of their own lives while also still being present for them, attentive to them, the mother of them.

NEGATIVITY BIAS

ALL HUMAN BEINGS ARE WIRED to place greater weight on negative events than on those that are positive or neutral. Evolutionarily, this negativity bias kept us safe by driving us to scan the horizon for threats, by committing to memory what locations or times of day were particularly risky to hunt or gather. Negativity bias is one of the basic ways our nervous systems try to keep us safe. But in the absence of saber-toothed tigers, perhaps we could let go of that bias a little.

When we become mothers, our negativity bias develops "roid rage." Our nervous systems run on hyperdrive to anticipate, root out, and destroy potential threats to our children. When my son was finally sleeping in his own room, I could hear his faintest cries—even if it was through two closed doors and a pair of earplugs—while my partner dozed peacefully.

The world can become an endless source of danger to the mother's hypervigilant nervous system. What can be missing is the capacity to discern irritants from catastrophes, bummers from disasters. And this lack of perspective can be directly or indirectly passed on to children in our constant refrain of "Careful…!" and "If you do that, you'll…" and "No, no, no." Not that these words aren't 100 percent essential at certain points, probably every day, but it's useful to know exactly when and what is called for.

Mothers who are conscious of their own negativity bias and are able to keep it in check by knowing when to let go can also pass on this discernment to their children to practice self-preservation without becoming afraid of the world, of others, and of themselves.

AMBIVALENCE

ONE OF THE MOST SHOCKING aspects of motherhood for me was the coexistence of diametrically opposed perspectives in my heart–mind. I could be dying for some time alone, some bodily separateness, but in the rare moments I got just that, I missed my child terribly—his smell, his physical presence, his raw vulnerability. While nursing, I was simultaneously wholly content and internally screaming to be anywhere else. Any time I had childcare, I was both giddy about my independence and wishing I could be a fly on the wall wherever he was. At work, I could finally have a continuous thought until the realization that I was separate from my child would break through my awareness, necessitating a refocus.

That's the thing about our complex and wondrous minds: we never think or feel just one thing. Yet it is often difficult for us to reconcile with multiple thoughts and feelings, especially if they seem to conflict. As Hamlet said, "There is nothing either good or bad, but thinking makes it so." Whether he was waxing philosophically or wishing for blissful ignorance is unclear, but what I do know is that thoughts are not inherently good or bad. It is our interpretation and judgment of them that puts them in one column or another. Without categorizing our thoughts as either positive or negative, therefore, they are all "just thoughts."

In meditation practice, when we notice we have gotten lost in our own minds, we label thoughts as "thinking"—not good thinking or bad thinking, just thinking. We gently and precisely observe whatever captured our attention and return our awareness to the feeling of the breath.

When we learn to regard all thoughts as just thoughts, we begin to see that the same applies to our emotions. We can label them and put them in jars called "good" or "bad," or we could just allow them to be, feel where they arise in our bodies, and expand to accommodate them.

I have learned to carry my ambivalence everywhere I go. Allowing my heart to swell with simultaneous joy and sadness, freedom and longing for togetherness, I open to the richness of my full experience. In the process, my compassion is deepened.

Motherhood is the ultimate practice in holding two (or more) seemingly conflicting truths simultaneously. Motherhood is the definitive "and" moment that teaches us to lean into the full catastrophe.

LESS HAPPY, MORE SATISFIED

MY BRILLIANT THERAPIST ONCE TOLD ME, in response to my agonizing over whether or not I wanted kids, that parents tend to be less happy but more satisfied with their lives. Since then, I have often found myself wondering which we truly long for. Is it happiness or is it satisfaction? Happiness seems so fleeting, so conditional and dependent on ever-shifting ground. Satisfaction, on the other hand, appears to possess more depth, richness, and meaning.

In so much of what we do, we strive for happiness. Whether it's how we eat (or don't), how we treat our bodies, how we buy, work, drink, smoke, have sex, much of what drives us has to do with attaining happiness. The number one marketing and advertising strategy on this planet could easily be reduced to "Buy this and find happiness." We spend much of our lives struggling for happiness, which often feels just out of reach. If we do manage a modicum, we might shift our attention to how to have more of it, how to hang on to it, how to remain in this positive state, all of which actually robs us of the experience of happiness in the moment. This makes me think that perhaps happiness is not ultimately what we are searching for.

Long before I became Buddhist, "contentment" was the word I associated with the philosophy. At the time, I interpreted the word as a detached state of calm, a means of removing myself from the grind of craving and aversion. What I have since learned, however, is that contentment—or what I think of as satisfaction—is about having perspective, gratitude, and a willingness not just to feel but to really move toward the full spectrum of experience.

This is motherhood. Sure, we have moments of happiness. Many of them. But they are not the be-all and end-all. It is the deep satisfaction of seeing our children grow and thrive and feeling ourselves change and attain deeper levels of compassion and wisdom that give our lives meaning, significance, and importance. Satisfaction is what makes the highs and lows doable and what allows us to feel like we have contributed something important to the world.

FINDING A SENSE OF HUMOR

THE DAY I PEED ON THE LIVING ROOM FLOOR, I did not find it funny. I had been trapped under my leisurely breastfeeder for what felt like hours, and my attempts at proper hydration betrayed me when my battle-scarred pelvic floor couldn't hold it in. I almost made it.

It took me a long time to come to terms with that moment of incontinence (not the only one by any stretch) because it signified some unanticipated loss of control, some truly ungraceful mother inadequacy. I told and retold the story in my attempts to process it, to find the humor in it. Eventually it became funny in the retelling, if only because by sharing it I opened up a break in my own veneer, one that let other moms own their own breaks, the funny–sad breaks that truly connect.

Tibetan Buddhist master Chögyam Trungpa said:

> It is impossible to overcome passion, aggression, and ignorance with a long face. We have to cheer up. When you begin to see yourself fully and thoroughly, then you discover your sense of humor. It is not the same as telling bad jokes. Humor here is natural joy, the joy of reality.

The joy of reality may feel counterintuitive for us as mothers, especially those of us who aspire to "get it together." Yet the path of motherhood provides endless opportunities to recognize the gritty, dear, messy, lovable parts of ourselves, our children, and our lives together.

Since peeing in the living room, I have aspired to recognize these moments as funny right when they happen, not just in the retelling. The countless spills, slime accidents, poop incidents, and discovering my son's "booger wall" have given me ample practice.

But in order to discover the humor in real time, I must be willing to accept the full mess—not just the funny but also the sad or angry, confused or scared. Finding the humor is not bypassing our experience but rather opening to the truth of its complexities.

OBSTACLES BECOME THE PATH

AS UNIVERSAL AS IS THE PATH of motherhood, we all experience it slightly differently. The age at which we become mothers, having one or two or more children, whether our work is paid or unpaid, whether our kids have special needs, whether we have a partner and how much that person is involved in raising children, our financial and social and educational circumstances—all these elements contribute to our unique experience of motherhood.

Our differences can also contribute to a sense of isolation, the feeling that no one is going through exactly what we are going through. And in a way this is true. In another way, however, all mothers are challenged to work with their unique circumstances through opening to what is, by working with their own minds, sensing into the minds and hearts of their children to guide and support them. Viewing what makes our experience of motherhood different from others through the lens of this common path can help us feel the collective spiritual importance of what we do.

Our unique circumstances also contribute to what we might interpret as a unique set of problems. Sibling dynamics, work–life balance, a "selectively incompetent" partner, poverty, so many societal systems stacked against us. Whatever the details, we face challenges based on the particulars of our lives. Given our specific set of problems, we approach our lives as projects, lining up what's not working and knocking them down one by one, if we are able.

The desire is to purify our lives by leaving problems behind us, removing them from our experience. But there is a different way.

One of my favorite mind-training slogans is "When the world is filled with evil, transform all mishaps into the path of bodhi." The most basic interpretation of this slogan is that whatever obstacles and challenges we face are not to be vanquished and left in our dust but rather to be ingested and metabolized so that they become the path. If we were weavers, our "evils" or difficulties on the path of motherhood would be woven into the fabric we are creating as seamlessly as our joys and our satisfaction. And the most basic definition of "evil" in this slogan, in my opinion, is the illusion that we are separate from one another.

By transforming all mishaps into the path of bodhi, we recognize obstacles as exactly what we need to work with. Granted we don't all encounter the same degree of obstacles, which range from "first-world problems" to serious issues. But the path is the same: work with them in their truest, simplest form. And in a radical and totally counterintuitive way, we can even begin to generate gratitude for our unique challenges because they keep us honest, sharp, and in the flow of our lives.

AWKWARDNESS

THE FIRST FEW DAYS AFTER my son was born were a flurry of attention and communal care. Family from near and far surrounded me and volunteered to hold, change, and soothe the baby while I slept or just caught my breath. But when the crowd dispersed and I assumed the majority of the moment-to-moment work of motherhood, I longed for company. I was forty when I gave birth and didn't know any other moms at the same age and stage as me, so I sought out a mom group, in part for diversion and in part for connection. What I found there, unfortunately, shared more parallels with middle school than with a welcoming assembly of similars (this was no fault of the other mothers who I'm sure were figuring out their own stuff in the moment).

Each time I left the group, I felt weird, wondering why I just didn't seem to fit in. I spent hours after interactions with the other moms replaying the ridiculous things I said, the ways they looked at me questioningly, wondering what they knew that I didn't. This awkwardness is by no means new and it did not begin with the birth of my son, but motherhood has amplified it a thousandfold.

The thing is, motherhood is intensely awkward. It's vulnerable and uncharted territory. We often don't know what the hell we're doing and might think that sets us apart because other moms have it all figured out. To the external observer, motherhood may appear to happen naturally, but when we are the ones doing it, it can feel strange and uncertain, kind of like doing "the robot" when a 1980s song comes on. We learn as we do. There is no other way. And that is damn awkward.

One approach that has helped me deal with my personal awkwardness and the awkwardness of motherhood is to stop being afraid of being a fool. When I let go of trying to hold it together, I find I am much more likely to be my genuine self, to laugh at my foibles, and to connect with other moms in theirs.

If we are lucky enough to find "our people"—those with whom we share a clear connection—motherhood may feel a little less awkward. Or, more realistically, we just lean into the awkwardness in good company. Whether we live in the same neighborhood, have kids about the same time, or rely on the same coffee shop for regular caffeine fixes matters less than having someone else—even just one person—who gets it.

THE TRUTH OF SUFFERING
(AKA THE TRUTH OF HAPPINESS)

IT IS REASONABLE TO ASSERT that we have an obsession with happiness. This goes beyond our natural human preference for pleasure over pain. There is a quality of trying to "win at life," as if we are playing a grand game of Space Invaders and life is bombarding us with endless challenges to either dodge or defeat while accumulating happiness points.

The realities of happiness and suffering are the basis for the Buddha's first formal teaching after he attained enlightenment, known as "the Four Noble Truths." The first is the truth of suffering—not "everything is terrible," but that some suffering in life is inevitable. We are born, we struggle, we get old (or don't), we may get sick, we die. Everything changes. Not everything goes our way. Eventually, we lose everyone and everything we love. These are the realities of living life in a human body.

The second Noble Truth holds that it is our resistance to the first Noble Truth that is the actual origin of suffering. Our craving for pleasure and aversion to pain is what makes these otherwise neutral phenomena positive or negative. The third Noble Truth is that there is a way out, a means of attaining freedom from the suffering that derives from our resistance to reality. And the fourth Noble Truth is the Noble Eightfold Path, the specific ways in which we train in nonattachment, nonresistance, and in working with reality.

What constitutes true happiness for a mother when working with the Four Noble Truths is different from what we might automatically think. As I release my grip on the idea of a life of ease one finger at a time, I find that happiness arises elsewhere: the gratitude experienced in filling out a review of systems before one of my son's doctor appointments and the awareness that so much about his body and overall health is working; the relief felt in apologizing to my child for wronging him; our shared celebration of accomplishments that are completely independent of me. The moments of our bodily connection, the spontaneous cuddles, unexpected "Mommy, I love you"s; the wise-beyond-his-years statements.

Even our suffering can feel useful, important, and poignant. It may not bring us happiness, per se, but a sense of clarity and understanding. We might reflect back to ourselves, *This is me living authentically. This is me not missing a moment of my real, messy, beautiful life.*

Our attempts to capture happiness with dualistic concepts of good or bad rob it of its complexity. They come from our deep discomfort with uncertainty, our need to see it to believe it, our reductionist and oversimplified understanding of life when we place that enormous "me" at its center. Once we move beyond this, we become capable of true bliss.

THE FIRST AND SECOND ARROW

SUFFERING IS BIG IN BUDDHISM. Admitting it exists, accepting it as inevitable, and committing to pay attention to it are in many ways the core of Buddhist philosophy and practice. This is shocking to our Western positive-affirmation-obsessed brains. We prefer to think that there is a way around suffering. With the right amount of money, the right house, spouse, city, job, body, diet, we can sidestep suffering and reside forever happily in la-la land.

Our first encounter with the first Noble Truth can be scary. "The truth of suffering" may sound as if all we can expect from life is doom and gloom. However, in reality the meaning is quite different. Inevitable suffering is sometimes the big painful milestones of loss and death but often it is just a nagging sense of *dis*-ease and unsatisfactoriness. Conceding this and accepting and feeling different forms of suffering surprisingly also gives us access to joy and delight. When we become less afraid of the full spectrum of our experience, we can live deep and authentic lives.

There is relief in admitting that some of the suffering in our lives is unavoidable. That means that there was never anything we could do to avoid it. No birthing plan, no sleep-training regimen, no approach to homeschooling in a pandemic could have saved us from that discomfort, whether it was a minor irritant or a true disaster. We learn that experiencing suffering is not an indication of "doing it wrong" but of simply living a human life.

It can also be helpful to discern the suffering that is inevitable from that over which we have a modicum of control. The natural unfolding of our lives in which there is constant change, disappointment, sadness, and a variety of emotions we experience as negative is the first arrow. It is how we respond to the first arrow that gives rise to or deflects the second arrow—the suffering of suffering.

The first arrow could be the tantrum your child threw in the checkout line, causing you to leave behind your full shopping cart, while the second arrow could be going down the mom-shame spiral. The first arrow could be a fight between you and your partner, while the second arrow could be "othering" yourself by imagining that other couples have it all figured out.

When we see the difference between the first and second arrows, we have a choice to make. Will we feel badly for feeling badly? Or will we seize that opportunity to practice radical acceptance and self-compassion?

CYCLES OF CLOSENESS

WHEN MY SON TURNED FIVE, it hit me hard. I mourned the end of his babyhood, even as I celebrated his new firsts: beginning to read, reaching the upper cabinets in the kitchen, his experiments with autonomy in moving farther and farther away physically and emotionally. Even as I celebrated his separations from me and his stretching into himself, I clung to the closeness I could, lying with him in bed as he fell asleep even though my partner felt it was "time" to let that go. Sometimes in the dark, his little hand would find mine, and my heart would clench with the desire to stop time. But these moments are precious precisely because they do not last.

Like any long-term relationship, the dynamic between ourselves and our children is not static. It is constantly shifting and changing. During pregnancy we live in the same body, eat the same food, breathe together. Our experiences overlap. From the moment of birth or adoption, we are constantly moving apart, then closer together, then further apart again. This can be felt most acutely when they start to explore their own bodies and environment independently, looking back over their shoulder to ensure we are still there but then returning to their investigations and discoveries.

These cycles of separation and closeness expand as our children age—the long arc is ultimately one of separation from a physical standpoint but potentially closeness emotionally. When they are youngest, the physical proximity is a given. They need what only our bodies can provide, literally and figuratively, to sustain them. They store up that sustenance and security to propel them into adulthood. The foundation in closeness we helped build gives them the confidence, judgment, and compassion essential to being a good human.

As mothers, we let go, then let go some more, and then even more. It is a heartbreak that is good and right. Trusting the cycles of closeness and separation and continuing to let go strengthens everyone involved.

TALKING TO OURSELVES

I MAY OR MAY NOT HAVE a tendency to overreact at times. I cannot say for sure, but my partner seems to think so. Once, after a disproportionately vehement reaction to something that turned out to be not so dire, I wrote myself a letter. In it, I shared the perspective I had gained on the other side of that overreaction. By providing some context and a more expansive view and suggesting how certain surrounding circumstances might have contributed to a lack of perspective, I offered myself the wisdom I realized would be helpful for the next time I lost it. I asked my partner to give me this letter when he saw history repeating itself.

This time-traveling fantasy is not original. Many writers have explored what they would tell their past or future selves. The wisdom in this exploration is to wonder aloud what we would say to ourselves in our worst moments when we have come through those circumstances and are stronger for it.

Perhaps the most powerful aspect of this exercise is simply relaying that no matter how difficult a moment is with our child, no matter how poorly they behaved or how badly we reacted, there is another side. This longer-term perspective has the potential to encourage us to stay with our experience even though we are in pain, desperate for relief, wishing the time away. Simply knowing that we do indeed make it to the other side inspires us to feel exactly what is arising and to be with it, expanding into the reaches of our emotional flexibility and deepening our compassion in the process.

Equally important, though, is the acknowledgment of a wise self who is somehow always there, even if her perspective is sometimes obscured by confusion. Creating lines of communications between our many "selves" offers us the opportunity to embrace our complexity, gradually viewing all aspects of our experience as just pieces of the puzzle.

TRUSTING OURSELVES

SO MUCH OF MOTHERHOOD is not knowing if you're doing it right. In 1946, Dr. Spock published the first parenting book. Over the course of the twentieth century, the number of parenting books exploded from that single one to thousands. With that came thousands of opinions about those books, their approaches, and their impact. While there is no shortage of the written word about how to mother, there is no actual formal preparation for this most important job. Where does that leave us?

In the midst of the pandemic, perhaps as a product of his age, temperament, and the months-long lockdown, my son began to have some behavioral issues. The seeds were already planted but this collision of factors really helped them blossom. His frustration intolerance, selective deafness, obsession with screen time, and physical outbursts gave my anxiety a new focal point. Like any self-respecting self-doubter, I took to the internet to consult Dr. Google and found no shortage of opinions on what was wrong. Soon I found myself speaking with a "parent whisperer," a child development specialist, and a pediatric occupational therapist who, in conducting our sessions virtually, turned my body into my son's sensory gym. During our third or fourth appointment, having been repeatedly body-slammed by him as I held a couch cushion and having logrolled across the floor clutching him to my body, I realized a few things:

> I love my child more than anything and will go to unimaginable lengths to support him.
> I will not intentionally harm my own body for his theoretical development.
> He will be okay.
> Yet again, I have had to pay experts a lot of money only to realize that I should trust my own judgment.

A mind-training slogan states, "Of the two witnesses, hold the principal one." In any situation, there are two perspectives: that of others and that which only you possess. This slogan guides us to trust ourselves, our judgment, and our basic goodness, even if that means messing it up sometimes. As universal as is the path of motherhood, we must each travel it on our own. All the parenting books, all the advice and opinions are fine, but in the end it comes down to you. You must decide what is best for you, your child, your family. No amount or quality of reassurance from others will feel satisfactory unless you know in your heart that you hold the principal witness. As we shift our allegiance from external sources of validation to our own, we build a sense of trust and confidence in our capabilities, even as we work with uncertainty, discomfort, and groundlessness.

JUST BECAUSE

THE MORNING BEFORE Christmas Eve 2020, I rolled out my yoga mat and, with a few minutes to spare, logged on to the 7:00 a.m. class with the small studio I'd practiced with for the duration of the pandemic.

While I waited for class to begin, my son came out of his room, and we had an ordinary first-thing-in-the-morning conversation. The only difference with this one was that the entire yoga class was able to listen in because I had not muted myself. Once I realized this and promptly muted myself, I reconstructed the conversation in my mind to imagine what the class had overheard:

ME: Good morning, my love. Did you pee pee?

HIM: Oh, I forgot. (*Leaves room, returns shortly, walks back over to me.*)

ME: Morning huggie?

HIM: (*Bends down to hug Lucy the cat first.*)

ME: Lucy gets the first hug. That's okay. I can wait.

HIM: Now you can have a huggie.

ME: I'm a little stinky this morning so be warned.

HIM: (*Leans his full weight into me, and we nuzzle one another's necks for a few moments.*) You smell pretty good to me.

ME: Thank you, my love.

HIM: Do I have school today?

ME: Yes, but it's from home. Do you want to come pick up the car with me later?

HIM: (*Excited.*) Okay! I guess we should go during one of my longer breaks.

ME: No, we'll need even more time than that. We can go after school is over and after my Mommy Sangha.

HIM: Okay. (*Goes and watches iPad while eating the banana I'd left for him.*)

ME: ...Did I not mute myself?! (*Hits Mute button.*)

I don't know if everyone listening could relate, but it was a moment of everyday intimacy we do not usually witness in others' lives. Or wish to share from our own. But the reality is that a lot of being a mother is just this: "Did you pee pee...Yes, you have school...Let's get the car later...Have a banana." The tiny invisible realities that make up life. I hope no one minded or that they took it in the spirit of a Mike Leigh film.

TRAIN IN THE THREE DIFFICULTIES

WHEN WE GET SWEPT UP in the momentum of daily life, we often fail to notice when our actions are out of sync with our underlying values. If pressed, we might list patience, affection, and compassion as priorities, while simultaneously our real lives reveal speediness, missed opportunities to connect, misinterpreting irritants as disasters. The only way we can recognize this inconsistency and begin to work with it directly and intentionally is to slow things down. Life is not about to slow down for us, so we have to take the first step. How we do that is messy and imperfect. That's the only way it could be.

"Train in the three difficulties" is a mind-training slogan about changing our habitual reactions. When we encounter challenges and obstacles, they usually catch us off guard. It may only be in retrospect that we realize we got hooked after all. I call this "mindfulness after the fact," but it is mindfulness in any case. The first of the three difficulties is recognizing this pattern earlier and earlier in the process by seeing ourselves in time and space, recognizing "Hey, I've been here before and I know where it leads me." When we see ourselves, we have choices. Practicing the first difficulty is essentially learning to see ourselves and lean in with non-judgmental curiosity.

The second difficulty is retracing our emotional steps to root out the origin of our habitual thoughts and actions. Where do they come from? What makes them more likely to emerge? Less likely? Usually this has to do with recognizing our attachment to pleasure, control, and knowing. Our entitlement to a life of ease. Our allergic reaction to discomfort. When we see where our habitual thoughts and actions originate, we can dig up that root ball and transfer it to the compost pile where it can nourish more productive actions.

The third difficulty is recognizing your mental and emotional "forks in the road" where you can either continue down habitual pathways or exert yourself as necessary to choose a different path. Neuroplasticity tells us that habitual pathways are more accessible; we keep thinking habitual thoughts and enacting habitual behaviors because it is easier for our brains to do so. But with awareness and commitment, we can see ourselves in action, interrupt the momentum of habit, and course correct. By practicing the three difficulties, we change, grow, and ultimately wake up.

ONE DAY WE WILL DIE

I'M DRAWN TO BUDDHISM for the same reason I love horror movies: both look directly at what we fear. Sickness, death, insanity, pain, and the inestimable unknown form the basis of every single horror movie I have ever seen, and I've seen a lot of them. Similarly, Buddhist philosophy doesn't just look at but leans into what we naturally abhor. Because none of us escapes death—that ultimate moment that comes too soon and without warning— Buddhist practice helps us prepare for it.

It's not just our ultimate death that we fear, as many of us can't even bring ourselves to think of that. Rather it is the tiny little deaths we face day in, day out that bring us anxiety and dread. Arguments, losses, and everyday disappointments. Our inability to stand in an elevator or on a subway train without breaking out our phones, as if moments without entertainment might actually kill us. Even boredom, allowing space and openness to exist when nothing in particular is happening, can be regarded unconsciously as a form of death.

The moment of death is as poignant and rich as the moment of birth. Beginning to view it as such makes it worthy of our attention. The more we pay attention, the more we come to know it and perhaps the less we have to fear it. I don't know if it is possible to not fear death. The idea of leaving all that is familiar, everyone I love, especially my child, is only outdone in terror by the idea of my child dying before me. But in facing its inevitability—accepting the truth of suffering and impermanence, knowing that one day it will all end—I can begin the peace process.

Ordinary experiences provide us with the training ground for working with the reality of death. We can practice preparing for our own death by witnessing and allowing the dissolution of any pleasant experience—a good meal, a beautiful day at the beach, the last day of vacation. Watch it as it begins to dissolve, noticing the knee-jerk desire to hold on tight, to fight the reality of its end. Recognizing our desire to hold on to pleasure and being willing to allow its natural ending helps us know what it's like to let go that final time.

SHOWING UP UNCONDITIONALLY

THE PATH OF MOTHERHOOD is ultimately one of showing up and staying unconditionally. That unconditionality extends to our children, ourselves, other mothers, our communities, and our planet. It also extends to the path of motherhood itself. We do not only show up when it goes our way; we do so in all its manifestations, twists and turns.

There are lots of parts of motherhood we may not like. In fact, allowing ourselves to dislike aspects of the path allows us to experience them with unconditional compassion and presence. Even as moods, momentary preferences, and superficial judgments ebb and flow, the commitment to showing up that we have for this experience and everyone touched by it only grows, deepening and expanding until we feel the interdependence of all beings in our bones.

This commitment to show up unconditionally is what ultimately makes motherhood the path to awakening. We have infinite opportunities to work with our minds, to let go of attachments and expectations, to expand into each moment fully, sensing and responding to the needs of our children, ourselves, and our environment. No other experience is as likely to bring us to our edge so regularly and then to push us over it again and again. As a result, we find that we are capable of more than we ever imagined. It is an honor and a privilege to walk the big, beautiful, messy path of motherhood. The mommysattva does so with openness, humor, and grace.

THE MOTHER'S
BODY

THE CLOCK STARTED TICKING for me at 8:20 a.m. the morning of July 27. After a forty-hour labor, the little nugget had shifted, descended, rotated, and made his long-awaited appearance, leaving my enormous, taut belly empty and flaccid. Until then, people told me, "You're carrying beautifully." Crossing the streets of New York City, strangers eyed my midsection and congratulated me because of how my baby bump grew forward instead of sideways: "Must be a boy, right?"

Toward the end of the pregnancy, though, the focus of strangers' comments began to shift to how my body should change. Giving birth became the starting gun—the moment I could concentrate on shrinking my belly, losing the baby weight, getting my body back. Breastfeeding became a diet aid, the stroller my treadmill.

The story of my body and my relationship with it has many chapters. In high school I was part awkward nerd, part stocky athlete, comforting myself with deep bowls of buttered pasta. As a nutrition graduate student, I measured day-to-day success by the ability to eat less than 1,200 calories. As a single working girl in my early thirties, I assuaged my insecurity by drinking too much wine, at times compensating by restricting calories and other times giving in to inevitable weight gain. Throughout each of these chapters, I was aware of my body as an object, a changeable thing to be manipulated depending on who was doing the looking.

When I got sober at thirty-three, I began the ongoing process of rebuilding trust in and with my body. In the years leading up to my pregnancy, I'd more fully embraced my body as it wanted to be—eating what I craved when I was hungry, stopping when I felt satisfied, and leaning into all the uncomfortable emotions that in the past had driven me to use alcohol and to manipulate food and my body. A month before I got pregnant, at my body's natural weight that included some new curves, my aunt thought I was already expecting.

When pregnancy took control of my body, I was mostly able to enjoy the ride. For forty weeks to the day, my body changed to accommodate the tiny human I carried and nourished from the inside, and each day I watched with wonder. Many mornings I stood naked in front of the bathroom mirror, caressing the profile of my growing tummy, staring at darkening nipples on heavy breasts, noticing the pads of fat that accumulated on my upper arms and outer thighs, and tracing the brown Magic Marker line from my breastbone down the middle of my stomach.

Even as time ground to a halt during my extended labor, I continued to watch as my body began the next stage of its brilliant metamorphosis. I marveled at how this vessel could continually adapt to the constant stream of changes: ultimately growing and nourishing a baby from the outside, reorganizing internal organs that had shifted to make room for him, and healing from the physical trauma of birth.

My stomach in particular held my fascination, from the early breastfeeding cramps that felt a lot like labor as my uterus resumed its original size and position to the days and nights of feeding my son as he rested comfortably on the soft ledge of my belly. Again I observed myself from all angles, first in the hospital bathroom and later at home during now-rare moments alone. I ran my hands down and around the calligraphic curves of my belly, which swung out to match the broadened lines of my breasts and hips. I wore my postpartum belly with pride on the walk home from the hospital in a fitted maxi dress. In the midst of August's swelter, I dressed for easy breastfeeding and to manage hormonal temperature fluctuations, not to minimize my prominent paunch. And when muscle memory brought my right hand to the place where I'd carried my son, I smiled to feel how its fullness endured though he no longer lived there.

Unfortunately, this pure affection for my postpartum belly didn't last long. My partner joked about awaiting the birth of our son's twin, and two male acquaintances commented that I still looked pregnant. Meanwhile, my inbox filled with tips on how to lose the baby weight. These jabs made me flush with shame and self-consciousness. I tried to suck my belly in, unsuccessfully, thanks to muscles that had stretched to their limit. I recalled with hot rage the common belief that women's bodies are supposed to snap back into place like rubber bands after birth. Those judgments—first from others and then again from myself—awakened something I thought I'd put to rest.

For the first few weeks of my son's life, whenever I awoke in the middle of the night to feed him, I was surprised when I looked down to see, illuminated by the streetlights, that broad, soft belly. If I fed him around other people, I tried to cover it with a burping cloth. Pushing the stroller, unearthing my prepregnancy clothes, meditating, having sex—there it was, not to be ignored. Though I could barely keep up with the caloric needs of breastfeeding, my mom belly persisted.

One day, as I was walking with my son along the East River, I listened to an episode called "The New You…It'll Do" on the podcast *The Longest Shortest Time*. I was struck by a comment from one of the guests, something like, "You can't grow a human being in your body and not be permanently changed by it." My immediate thought was "Of course I can't!"

Meanwhile, my son grew stronger. Sometimes after eating, he would stretch his legs and, using my belly as support, try to stand. When he'd take a break and we'd gaze into each other's eyes, I'd squish his tiny belly to see how it wrinkled and creased and engulfed the hollow of his navel. Then looking down at my own belly, I realized how similarly it moved. How could I love one and not the other?

I began to see my belly through different eyes: beautiful and complete. An adaptable instrument that facilitated movement and play, not an object to be chiseled and critiqued. Again my hands found my belly and touched it with a sense of gratitude and love. I stopped sucking it in, got rid of the clothes that made it feel uncomfortable, and embraced how other clothes accommodated this new curve.

Ticking clocks, mom jeans, MILFs, the mom pooch. Few bodies are under the microscope as intensely as those of mothers. They should be soft but not fat. Warm and welcoming but not overly solicitous. There is a special place in hell for people who target the mother's body as a site for continual improvement. As if we don't have enough reasons to question whether we are good enough, the pressure on moms to recapture their prepregnancy physique steamrolls over the fact that their miraculous bodies have just generated another human being.

Women are used to walking the tightrope of society's judgments about their bodies, and that balancing act grows more precarious in motherhood. Like the path of motherhood itself, the mother's body is ours to reclaim. To elevate to the sacred. It is our job to smash the ways in which our bodies have been limited by the patriarchy and establish our own definition of a mother's body. To infuse our relationship with our bodies with gentleness, kindness, compassion, and reverence. Changing our relationship with our bodies begins as an inside job and spreads outward as each of us feels entitled to claim our power. Our own body sovereignty. Society's demands on the mother's body are a wolf in sheep's clothing, not what they seem. Not the truth. They are the oversimplification of what cannot be contained. How we hold our minds and hearts determines whether we view our bodies as limited and in need of repair, or miraculous, powerful, and innately good.

THE MOTHER'S BODY IS BASICALLY GOOD

FEW RELATIONSHIPS ARE AS COMPLICATED as a woman's relationship with her own body: this thing that has been with her since before birth, this thing that has changed so much, endured so much, that adapts to so much, and yet is so often seen as inadequate, in need of improvement.

Becoming a mother has the potential to radically shift a woman's relationship with her body. Instead of evolving over the course of years, the adaptations and accommodations of the mother's body during pregnancy—demonstrations of its pure instinct and intelligence—happen over a much shorter span of time, literally changing from one day to the next. Mothers who adopt also experience this radical shift in their bodies, differently but no less significantly, as their bodies become the vehicle of caregiving. As a result, a woman has the opportunity to sit back and enjoy the ride if she holds her mind a certain way.

All beings possess "basic goodness," an inherent and enduring quality that is unchanged by time. Basic goodness is likened to a jewel that has been buried underground. It is a rare and beautiful thing that must be unearthed by working with our confusion, and it never loses its value. It remains unconditionally pure and perfect at all times.

Extending the definition of basic goodness to include her body, a mother radically changes the soundtrack playing in her mind. Rather than being defined by harsh external criticism, judgments, and impossible standards, how she feels about her body—how she feeds it, moves it, cares for it—can be driven by a deep and abiding internal sense of wisdom, confidence, and trust. By consistently sensing inward, a mother is able to interpret what her body is communicating in real time, to understand what is needed, and to take action to meet her own needs, constantly working with the confusion that comes from conflicting external views.

EXPANDING TO ACCOMMODATE

A MOMMYSATTVA'S JOB in working with things as they are is to meet whatever comes her way and change accordingly. The mother's body can show her the way. It is constantly adapting, expanding, and accommodating, both literally and figuratively.

Beginning with pregnancy and continuing for the rest of her life, the mother's body is responding to changes that are physical, neurological, and psychological. From the moment of conception, bones and organs shift to prepare for pregnancy and birth, then resume some approximation of their prepregnancy position. The mother's senses sharpen irreversibly to the needs of her child. Psychologically, she is forever changed—now attuned to and completely responsible for two bodies instead of one.

Our meditation practice and underlying view of basic goodness allow us to see how the mother's body continues to adjust and allow. It is the master adapter. Like all bodies, the mother's body is always in the present moment; it is incapable of existing in the past or future. The mind is not always so reliable, whether dwelling in the past, shooting forward into the future, or simply worrying, anticipating, wishing, hoping. From the stability of the ever-adapting body, the mommysattva is encouraged to come back to the present moment, to expand to accommodate exactly what is happening right now.

THE ORIGIN OF ALL THINGS

THE FEMALE ANATOMY IS SO OFTEN the target of disdain, disgust, even hatred. I have often wondered how this could be when it is literally the origin of us all. This epic disconnect confuses us as girls (and encourages misogyny in boys as well as in girls), when we learn to cover up, keep our legs together, defend our pelvic area, alter the appearance of our pubic hair, hide our periods, deodorize our natural smells. Then if we become pregnant, we are suddenly celebrated for the same parts that were previously shrouded in shame. If we are unable to become pregnant, we are shamed for our bodies not doing "what they are supposed to do."

One morning, as I was rising from the toilet—of course the bathroom door was wide open and my little guy was there keeping me company—my son exclaimed, "Ewwwww," at the sight of my vulva. I seized the moment to nip that familiar critique of the female anatomy in the bud: "Let me tell you something about this. This is my vagina, the place you came out of. My body took one cell from daddy and then grew you and pushed you out through here. So that thing you are saying 'Ewwwww' to is where everything and everyone comes from, and it is magical. It may seem weird that pee and blood and poop come out of here but that comes along with my body's ability to create you." My son stood stunned at this revelation. I wondered if I'd overdone it, but then he exhaled a long "Wow."

My proud ownership of my anatomy has been hard won. Like most women, I have struggled with shame about my vagina being "too wet" or "too dry." I have bemoaned its cycles and their accompanying pain, inconvenience, and expense. I have lamented how it makes me vulnerable in a way that a biologically male body is not. Becoming a mother helped me dress down my shame and embrace this miraculous part that gave me my favorite person.

Weeks after the little "lesson" with my son in the bathroom, we were visiting my parents. He was playing soccer in the front yard with my mom when they got to talking about the day he was born. I later learned that he seized this opportunity to educate my mom about where he came from. When she recounted the story to me later, she parroted my son: "Those vaginas are ah-mazing."

GETTING YOUR BODY BACK

A PAINFUL PHRASE MANY NEW MOTHERS hear is about "getting your body back," as if in giving birth a body is lost rather than gained. For me those unsolicited comments came during my last trimester, when I was completely reveling in my new body. To reduce the pregnant mother's body in this way, to an object that must be recaptured, is terribly demeaning. It suggests that the most valuable aspect of that body is how it appears from the outside, and that any evidence of this momentous transformation it has undergone must be erased from view.

Similarly, as we were neck-deep in the coronavirus pandemic, many people voiced their desire for things to get back to normal, even though in a literal sense that would mean returning to collective ignorance in terms of rampant systemic racism, the extreme vulnerability of many populations, the lack of equity in health care, financial resources, and social supports. Not unlike matrescence, the pandemic involved a period of destabilization and reorganization on many levels. The accompanying uncertainty made many of us so uncomfortable we would have preferred going back to the bad old days instead of accepting that we would be forever changed by what had happened.

You cannot go back in time. And why would you want to? Everything we encounter in our lives becomes part of our path. The pandemic forever changed our awareness and allowed us to see ourselves more clearly. Becoming a mother forever changes our bodies in ways we cannot begin to grasp. We are in the middle of a massive societal recalibration the results of which will only become clear in time. The same applies to our evolving perspectives on our bodies.

The mind of meditation tells us that there is no past body to lament, no future body to become attached to. We have just the present-moment body exactly as it is, influenced by past events but not beholden to them. How we treat that body might somehow influence how it manifests in the future, but that outcome is not under our control.

It is not possible to recapture a body that you had in the past or to finally "achieve" the ideal body you never had before becoming a mother. It is possible, however, to rediscover your body every day. Every moment. To accept it as it is, even if you aren't fully comfortable with it. Even if at times you don't like it very much. Even with ambivalence, we can respect our bodies, care for them, relieve their discomfort, meet their needs.

As with any long-term relationship, the one you have with your body can never return to a former phase. It can, however, deepen, sweeten, become more subtle and expansive. This is the body you were born with and the one you will die with. How will you treat it?

POWER AND VULNERABILITY

IF YOU HAVE NEVER DONE goddess pose in yoga, let me try to explain it. Facing the long line of your yoga mat, you step out sideways into a wide straddle. With the toes pointed outward, bending your knees to ninety degrees directly over your feet, you are standing in a wide-open squat. Your arms are also held wide with elbows at right angles, hands active.

The pose is powerful. By engaging nearly every muscle group in the body, it is as if the yogini were spring-loaded, catlike, ready to pounce. It is also vulnerable, with every part of the body exposed and open.

According to Western ideals, goddess pose is quite unfeminine. It is designed to take up space, a radical concept for women who are taught that femininity equals smallness. It is sprawling, brash, and unapologetic. Women who are educated from a young age to protect their pelvic area because of its vulnerability to violation might initially be surprised at how they are opening their knees in a position of confidence and authority.

Goddess pose is an ideal metaphor for the mother's body: open, powerful, vulnerable, capable, expansive. Assuming this pose, inside or outside of a formal yoga practice, connects us with the basic goodness of our bodies. We may not love every aspect of our bodies, but in taking goddess pose we acknowledge their inherent and formidable might.

THE BODY AS INSTRUMENT

OUR CULTURE, MORE OFTEN THAN NOT, emphasizes the importance of our bodies as objects that exist for the viewing pleasure of others. How our bodies look from the outside matters more than what they do, how they adapt to changing circumstances, how they transform over time.

The appearance of our bodies, as much as advertising and marketing efforts would have us believe otherwise, is largely out of our control. Their size and shape, our facial structure, hair texture, how close or far we are from that idolized minority—these characteristics are governed by genetics. We could spend decades and fortunes trying to distance ourselves from that heritage, but our efforts would not only be in vain but also in denial of our lineage and our diversity.

Instead, the vantage point on our bodies can be shifted from external to internal by focusing on what the body does and how it feels. This is actually a much more nurturing and compassionate view of our bodies, and one we can carry with us to the moment of our death.

The mother's body is an incredible instrument. Of course the capacity for pregnancy is miraculous, but no matter your route to motherhood, your body is your primary tool of caregiving, modeling, and presence for your children. From skin-to-skin contact, early feedings, playing, cuddling, and beyond, it is our bodies that enact our presence.

Australian coach, meditation teacher, and Mommy Sangha member Fiona describes how when her daughter experiences night terrors, the only thing she can do is to comfort her with her body. Holding her daughter, holding the space, sharing the ride is what she can offer when there is nothing else. To provide that safety and steadfastness may not feel like much when our children are suffering but it communicates volumes: *Yes, you are suffering and I wish I could take that from you, but I cannot, and so I will be here with and for you with my very being, this physical manifestation of my love for you.*

The shift from viewing your body as an object to seeing it as an instrument takes time and practice. Whenever you find yourself looking at your body from the outside, critically, judgmentally, with an editing eye, notice this, recognize the confusion, and redirect your attention to inhabiting the body, feeling it from the inside. The process of becoming a mother provides endless opportunities to connect with the body—how it feels, how it performs, how it shows up moment to moment. The practice of shifting our allegiance from an outside-looking-in perspective to an embodied one defines our relationship as one of devotion, unconditional love, and gratitude.

THE INTELLIGENCE OF THE BODY

OUR CULTURE MAKES IT DIFFICULT to grasp the idea of an innately intelligent body. The pervasive view in our culture is that the body must be directed, overpowered, manipulated, and managed for optimal functioning. When we subscribe to this view, however, we discount the myriad ways in which the body self-regulates, naturally adapting to the constant changes that affect it. Often, we focus on a narrow slice of the pie—our appearance—thereby negating the majority of what our bodies do all by themselves.

Consider all the ways the body functions to care for and protect us. All the involuntary activities it is constantly engaged in—circulation, respiration, detox and elimination, ovulation and menstruation, the brain presiding over all. Consider how the body signals danger through the experience of pain. How it alters its metabolization of nutrients depending on whether we are getting too much or not enough. How it takes a single sperm cell and instinctively grows and nourishes a human body inside our own.

The innate intelligence of our bodies is inextricable from the fact that they are always in the present moment. Because they are always in the present moment, whatever they do is in response to what is actually happening.

In meditation practice, when we align the mind with the present-moment body, we reconnect with our innate intelligence. We reconnect with the capacity to sense and respond to events in real time. We connect to this vessel that knows—has always known—what it is doing.

SUFFERING AND THE BODY

RIGHT BEFORE MY SON TURNED ONE, a series of unfortunate events unfolded in my life. My body and mind were stressed, exhausted, and had simply exceeded their capacity, but rather than allow myself to slow down and turn toward these realities, I continued to push myself, strapping his growing body to my chest in a front carrier and exceeding my limits, physically and emotionally. Because I didn't heed the warnings of pain my body was sending me, I herniated a cervical disc and inflicted permanent damage on my spine. On his first birthday, I couldn't even pick him up. I stopped breastfeeding abruptly so that I could take something for the pain while I awaited surgery.

None of the painkillers worked for me. The only place I found temporary relief was in the pool, standing in water up to my chin so that my spine could elongate, finally relieving the compression at the source of my agony. At night I tossed and turned, desperately trying to find a position that would provide relief, but there was none. Ultimately, I learned to relax into the pain. I realized that my resistance to it, my bracing against it, only distorted and amplified it. In relaxing into my pain, I experienced the raw searing sensation that was there—nothing more and nothing less. And it sucked!

This experience radically changed my understanding of suffering and the body. Walking around New York City, I looked at people differently. All these people with human bodies that experience pain, injury, and illness. I saw their distress, their natural resistance and aversion to discomfort, and how it ultimately only increased their suffering. I also saw people whose norm was pain and disability and began to see how that changes everything.

Part of what makes it so difficult to consistently connect with our present-moment bodies is their capacity for suffering. Our bodies hurt. They experience illness and injury. Some of us live with pain, disease, and disability every day of our lives. Ultimately, our bodies grow old (if we're lucky) and eventually we die. As with all things, what we resist persists. The suffering we experience in the body is much like the suffering we experience in our hearts and minds. When we resist it, it becomes amplified and distorted. If we were able to turn toward our suffering, we would experience it purely—nothing more and nothing less.

To change our relationship with the suffering of our bodies, we might start to view it as a form of communication. Our bodies are constantly telling us what is up, from signaling our need to pee (like, all the time) to flagging our hunger to quite unmistakably screaming at us that we have reached some edge in terms of pain to communicating we absolutely must rest. Framing our suffering as our body's means of communicating with us can soften our reaction; we can develop gratitude for this information and this opportunity to do something different, whether that something is in the form of relief or simply paying attention.

DESIRE

WHEN A WOMAN BECOMES A MOTHER, she may be expected to let go of any desires for her own pleasure and satisfaction and place the needs of her children before her own. Yet those desires remain.

A mother is a human first—wired for pleasure, desiring of sensation and experience. A woman's desire—her craving for pleasures from food, love, work, creativity, sex, beauty, and experience—is the subject of inordinate judgment and surveillance. A mother's appetite for sensation becomes something that she learns to contain, measure, and hide.

In some ways, our desire can signal craving or addiction—the subtle intolerance to discomfort that causes us to seek out pleasurable distraction. We can identify this type of desire by noticing what it is in reaction to, by staying with the body as the urge for food or wine or acquisitions washes over us, thrilling our brains with the possibility of relieving our suffering. If and when we pull the trigger and partake of these pleasures, we can ride the arc of anticipation, consummation, and, inevitably, dissolution. While it is natural to experience sadness at the end of a pleasurable experience, the feelings of loss and confusion as an experience ends may be a sign that we thought it was "the thing" that would finally save us. We are surprised to find ourselves unchanged, our suffering unmitigated after the experience is over. Then we start hunting for the next fix.

In other ways, our desire is a manifestation of our living, breathing, dynamic bodies constantly interacting with the world. We were born with these incredible senses that allow us to taste, hear, feel, smell, and see our way through our lives. To simply write off desire as "attachment" denies the wisdom with which our bodies engage with the world: playfully and viscerally.

How do we discover a middle way in working with desire? How do we allow ourselves to live richly and sensually without self-medicating or spiritually bypassing our appetites? By paying attention, remaining embodied, and staying receptive to the constant stream of communication from our bodies. As a result, we might even realize that our desires extend beyond the boundaries set for us by our culture and finally discover what fulfills and excites us.

FOOD

A WOMAN'S RELATIONSHIP WITH FOOD may be fraught long before she becomes a mother. Once she is charged with the care and feeding of a little one, that relationship can grow even more complex. From imperfectly evidenced food restrictions during pregnancy to early urgings to "lose the baby weight" to the bites of cold mac 'n' cheese surreptitiously consumed standing over the kitchen sink, it can be difficult for a mother to prioritize feeding her own body regularly and satisfyingly, without fear, shame, or anxiety.

The mother's body is basically good. Like all human bodies, it must get the basics of safety, sleep, water, and food to simply function. But eating is not just about meeting those most basic needs. Our bodies are hardwired to derive pleasure from food. Our taste buds and the signals they send our brains are an evolutionary benefit that have kept us alive, not to mention contributed to a world of sensuality around flavor, temperature, and textural combinations. Bringing attention to the mother's relationship with food, therefore, is an act of working with her body and her very humanity exactly as it is.

As with all things, when we work against ourselves, there are consequences. When we ignore difficult emotions, they become amplified and distorted only to cause us more suffering in the future. Similarly, when we work against our bodies—denying ourselves the quantity and quality of food that would provide satisfaction—there is a backlash. When we give our bodies inadequate food, our physiology's protective countermeasures kick in, causing us to seek it out in chaotic ways. When we don't give ourselves permission to eat the foods we like, we ultimately find ourselves bingeing on those very things.

Working with our bodies, on the other hand—allowing our bodies and our appetite to be as they are, just as we do in meditation practice—ends the battle with ourselves, drops the tension created by arbitrary restrictions, and sharpens our awareness of what, when, and how much we need to eat to experience true satisfaction.

BODY IMAGE

A MOTHER'S RELATIONSHIP WITH HER BODY sets the tone for so much of what a daughter or son absorbs. When that relationship is one of respect, accommodation, and communication, children learn to work with—not against—their bodies, to listen to what they are telling them, to interpret that information in real time, and to respond as best as they can.

A positive body image is not always feeling positively about your body. We all have bad body image days (even those of us who work in this space and are considered "body image experts"). Rather, having a positive body image implies there is a constant receptivity to our bodies; we give ourselves permission to feel however we are feeling—whether that be pleasure and comfort or pain and sadness—and consistently meet the body's needs day after day, even as they continue to change.

When a mother's relationship with her body is one of battle, denial, and manipulation—restricting what we eat, exercising for the purposes of remodeling our bodies, verbally denigrating our bodies to deny their inherent worthiness, suggesting that we become deserving of love and acceptance only when we achieve some future status of body control and mastery—the message is decidedly different: the body is dangerous, not to be trusted.

It is unsurprising that many of us have such an adversarial relationship with our bodies. We are taught from an early age that we simply cannot trust these vessels we walk around in. Thus our beliefs, thoughts, and actions are driven by anticipatory anxiety and the universal wish to live in bodies regarded as acceptable by society. This distorts our natural capacity for self-regulation, the ability to introspect and discern what we are feeling moment to moment and what we truly need to feel safe, satisfied, and cared for.

Cultivating a positive body image is possible only through trust in our innate intelligence, attention to the ongoing communication process, and a willingness to consistently meet our basic human needs. It may not be a smooth or straightforward process at times, but it is essential to feeling at home in our bodies.

SELF-CARE

I GREW UP IN THE ERA OF "Calgon, take me away." These days, "self-care" is all about the salt scrubs and lavender pillow spray. The industries of self-care have a deep and abiding love for mothers, or at least for their money. Advertising and marketing efforts target mothers with various products and services that supposedly amount to self-care. Hair, skin, and nail products. Spa services. Bath products in particular are an apparent boon to mothers, on the one hand acknowledging how even our most basic acts of hygiene are affected by motherhood while on the other suggesting that taking a shower is some kind of luxury.

Does the commercialization of self-care really point to what product or service we need to acquire? Or is true self-care subtler, perhaps not even something for which we need to shell out dollars? I love a good bath or skin care product, believe me, but what I have come to see as true self-care cannot be purchased.

Acts of self-reverence. Self-respect. Self-devotion. That is caring for the self. Saying no. Picking up the phone. Not picking up the phone. Taking a nap. Creating and defending boundaries. Social media breaks. Asking myself what I need in this moment. Accepting help. Giving myself permission to feel whatever it is I am feeling.

These are the deeper and more nuanced actions we can take to ensure our safety, sanity, and preservation. These are the steps that no one else can take but ourselves because no one else understands what is unfolding for each of us in any given moment and what is truly needed.

BODY GRATITUDE

OUR NEGATIVITY BIAS, especially in the context of our self-aggressive and problem-solving culture, causes us to focus on what doesn't work about our bodies rather than what does. A radical practice, therefore, is to have body gratitude. Intentional, continual body gratitude that acknowledges and appreciates what our bodies do for us and what does work, and on which we intentionally choose to focus:

I am grateful for this body that is my primary instrument of caregiving for my child(ren).

I am grateful for this body that serves as my child's home base.

I am grateful for these strong legs that carry me everywhere I go.

I am grateful for these arms that can encircle and embrace my child.

I am grateful for this body that can dance in the living room.

I am grateful for this body that can run, walk, do yoga, ride a bike.

I am grateful for these eyes, nose, ears, mouth, and skin that let me experience the world sensually.

I am grateful that I don't have to control my lungs' breathing, my heart's beating.

I am grateful that I have never had to think about my pancreas or spleen (if you have, perhaps you could focus on how your body has adjusted to whatever parts are not working perfectly).

I am grateful for my clitoris whose only job is to give me pleasure!

I am grateful for all the processes my body is engaged in that I have never even considered.

A body gratitude practice is not meant to squash negative feelings about our bodies. We cannot heal self-aggression with self-aggression, and rendering certain thoughts off limits is unkind and unrealistic. We can, however, broaden our perspective so that we are taking in the full picture—acknowledging that in addition to what causes us distress, there is much to be grateful for.

EVERY CHILD
IS A BUDDHA

MUCH OF THE PARENTING ADVICE available to us is about how to make our own lives easier. Obviously written from the parent's point of view—how could it be otherwise?—we are most concerned with how to triage parenting's inevitable difficulties, how to do it right, and how to find balance in our own lives. It's wonderful that so much of the discourse is intended to support mothers, and yet so often missing from the parenting books and the TED talks is real compassion for our children.

My teacher Susan Piver describes how in relationships we operate with "projectors" on our foreheads. We shine those projectors on potential mates and mentally attempt to bend them to our will based on the hopes, dreams, and expectations we have accumulated over the course of our lives. Conflict inevitably arises when that person fails to perform as expected.

The same could be said for how we project on to our children. Many of us anticipate that motherhood will look and feel a certain way. We envision our children will have all the qualities and characteristics we prize and none of the ones we fear. We might imagine that it is our role to ensure they develop accordingly. Some of this wishful thinking is directly related to a life of ease for ourselves—and who doesn't want that? Other wishful thoughts are consciously or unconsciously born of the desire for a life of ease for our child. But is this sculpting and editing of our children truly our job?

Jon and Myla Kabat-Zinn introduced the concept of a child's sovereignty in their book *Everyday Blessings: The Inner Work of Mindful Parenting*: "In honoring our children's sovereignty, we make it possible for them to do two things: show themselves as their 'true seeming,' and find their own way." The word "sovereignty" gave shape to something I had been contemplating long before I was pregnant: that my most important role besides keeping my child safe was to help him become exactly who he (she? they?) is. The fundamental belief inherent in honoring a child's sovereignty is that we should all be supported to become authentically who we are because that is inherently good.

Every child needs emotional connection and security. To be treated with dignity and respect. They need to know where they fit in. The family is their first and most basic form of society; it provides the context for the greater society as they grow into themselves. The mommysattva, who knows her child better than anyone, is uniquely poised to guide them through this process, maintaining intact their sovereignty and their true "Buddha-nature."

BUDDHA-NATURE

WE ALL HAVE BUDDHA-NATURE. Sometimes translated as "basic goodness," Buddha-nature is the clear, intelligent, inherently whole, already enlightened quality that every being possesses, even though it is often obscured by confusion. Commonly used analogies for Buddha-nature include the blue sky that exists even when concealed behind the clouds, the lotus that rises unscathed from the muck, a jewel that must be uncovered from where it has been buried.

Our children are born with Buddha-nature; it is not something they must earn or accumulate. We see it in everything they do and everything they are—when they touch the petals of a flower, when they experience the heartbreak of losing a favorite toy, when they realize for the first time the power in the words "I love you" and "I hate you."

It may be easier to see the Buddha-nature of our kids when they are agreeable or very young and more difficult as they grow increasingly complex, as they grapple with the pain of being human, as they bump up against their own confusion. But their Buddha-nature does not waver. We can remind ourselves that throughout all their ups and downs, our child is always Buddha. She might be angry Buddha one moment and anxious Buddha the next. He could be clingy Buddha in the morning and hyper-active Buddha in the afternoon. They might alternate between revelatory Buddha, purely joyous Buddha, wise-beyond-their-years Buddha, and affectionate Buddha. But they are always Buddha.

ATTENTION IS THE
MOST BASIC FORM OF LOVE

OUR CHILDREN DO NOT NEED to get everything they want in order to feel loved. Quite the opposite. It is in our willingness to not always appease them that we demonstrate our true love. It is much more generous to pay genuine attention to our children so that they learn what it is to be human. That sometimes they will get what they want while other times they will get what they need. That difficulty is worth experiencing directly: there is a place for being considerate, compassionate, and kind, as well as for pursuing personal desires and curiosities.

John Tarrant Roshi has said, and I have come to believe this in my bones, "Attention is the most basic form of love; through it we bless and are blessed." By paying attention with our bodies, hearts, and minds and discerning moment to moment what is needed by this child standing in front of us, this is how we love them. It is not always the easiest path. There is conflict and disagreement and pain. But the intention is love. The impact is love.

THE HEIGHT OF GENEROSITY

OUR KIDS ARE MADE UP of constellations of characteristics. Some are easier to accept than others. What helps us practice the generosity of allowing our children to be who they truly are is realizing that we cannot pick and choose their qualities according to what feels easiest or most desirable. To know that his deep sensitivity and empathy is packaged alongside his hyperresponsivity to perceived criticism. That her easygoing nature is packaged alongside the seeming inability to follow specific directions. That their deep curiosity is packaged alongside their endless need to test limits. The critical question when it comes to these constellations is "Can I accept, love, and nurture the whole package?"

It is the height of generosity to allow our children to be exactly who they are. This is only amplified when practiced by the mommysattva, who not only allows her child to be who they are but assists them in cultivating these qualities and working with themselves in an ongoing way, reflecting back to them where leaning into their discomfort might actually be the path to realization. Each of us is vulnerable to the idea that we can pick and choose our desirable qualities. The mommysattva, understanding the value of the whole package, can guide her children to expand to accommodate their own wholeness.

WHEN OUR KIDS
ARE AT THEIR WORST

ALONGSIDE MY ROLE IN SUPPORTING my son to be exactly who he is, I committed to making it clear that my love for him never wavers—in fact, it only grows—in his most difficult moments. During a nuclear meltdown, when he explodes in a fit of rage, when he goes for the jugular ("You are the worst mommy in the world" or "I hate your cooking"), my love remains constant and unconditional.

We cannot underestimate the importance of communicating this fact to them explicitly. As they are breaking down—when they are at their most volatile and vulnerable—imagine the impact of knowing that they are held and safe and that we will ride the rollercoaster with them no matter where it takes us. Of knowing that it is human to break, that there are no emotions that are off limits (even if not all behaviors in response to those emotions are okay), that it is safe to learn how to deal with pain, disappointment, and suffering in real time with us.

BEWARE THE OVERLY COMPLIANT CHILD

OUR JOB AS MOTHERS is to encourage and support our children to become exactly who they are, while also helping them learn to exist in community, to be sensitive to the different needs and experiences of others without living for others. When children feel that this is the quality of our love and support, they are free to grow into the individuals they were meant to be.

This is not always going to be easy. Between the terrible twos, threenagers, the fearsome (or fucking) fours—and I don't even know what I'll do with an actual teenager—it's clear that the ages our children move through are associated with difficult behaviors. These behaviors make our lives as mothers challenging at best. But part of why we perceive these behaviors as challenging is due to our expectation that children should be easy, that their behaviors must comply with our expectations, that they should make life a smooth ride.

I have come to see my son's difficult behaviors through every age and stage as him doing his job. That job evolves and becomes more nuanced over time, but at its heart it involves him learning, figuring life out, stretching into his autonomy. When my son is particularly agreeable, I find myself wondering what's at play: is he in a moment of balance, contentment, and connection, or is he bending to what he imagines are my wishes? When is that okay and when should it be otherwise? I often take those opportunities to state in no uncertain terms how much I love him, both when we are sharing peaceful, happy moments and when we disagree, argue, and struggle. This seems to allow him to ride the different energies of his authentic self instead of shaping his behaviors in reaction to (or anticipation of) my needs.

COOPERATION OR COERCION?

WHEN MY SON WAS THREE and honing his ability to test my limits, I developed my 1-2-3 method (I know, very original). He knew that once I started counting, he needed to do what I had asked before I got to three, at which point consequences would be imposed. I lived in fear of the day that he realized the consequences weren't actually so dire. But he also lived in fear: even if the consequences were only a few minutes less on his iPad, being "punished" was excruciating for him. Whereas my method worked at first in terms of getting him to do what I wanted, as he got a bit older it gradually assumed a different cast.

One night at shower time—which can be exasperating after a long day—he was procrastinating in his usual fashion when I started to slowly count to three. When I got to two, I didn't realize that he was in the kitchen getting undressed and was trying to comply with my request. There, as he heard me say the number two, he disintegrated with the fear of consequences and confusion at my continuing to count while he was doing what I asked. He screamed in protest, and it was many seemingly endless minutes before we were able to piece together what had just happened.

When I understood, I was leveled. It felt abusive. I was terrorizing him. This was not how to teach him to listen and cooperate. And it certainly did not make for a smooth transition into bedtime. What was a handy trick when he was three years old became a way of controlling him when he was capable of more understanding and cooperation.

I owned it. Looking into his eyes as tears rolled down his cheeks, I apologized to him and told him that what I had just done was unfair. What I did not say was that I realized how I had betrayed his trust, changed the rules without warning, and gone from being collaborative to being controlling. I promised myself in that moment that I would find another way of working with him that met both our needs. (I'm still working on this.)

At times it is necessary to impose our will. Whenever safety is concerned or when behavior has become extreme—harmful to themselves or others—we must act immediately and unilaterally, and deal with hurt feelings later. But what I am learning is that my child is capable of solving problems alongside me—when I know how to engage him. So quickly has he evolved from the simple being whose needs were food, sleep, or a clean diaper to a much more complex one who is in many ways unknown to me. I continue to know my child by engaging him fully as a human being, by trying to understand his perception of our shared situations, and by finding solutions that are not only aligned with my needs but also respectful of his.

BAD BEHAVIOR

DEALING WITH BAD BEHAVIOR is a fact of motherhood—a difficult one that has sometimes caused me to question whether I really "like" the true work of parenting at all. Discerning whether behavior is age-appropriate limit testing or evidence of something else; recognizing and not perpetuating power struggles; turning fully toward what our children, their behavior, and even our own limitations are demanding: this is some of the most difficult work we ever do.

A child's job is to individuate, to test limits, to understand how and where they fit into the social fabric, beginning with the microcosm of their own families. Sometimes (maybe often) this means behaving in ways we consider negative, inappropriate, or in need of correction.

To deal with bad behavior while also protecting our children's sovereignty, we must confront our own confusion. We must recognize what is beneath a desire to "power over" our children—to maintain control, to make our lives easier—and what lies beneath a tendency to "power under" them—to avoid conflict, be the parent–buddy. Finding the middle way allows us to share power *with* our children so that we collaborate to solve problems and they ultimately become their own guiding voice.

Children, like all of us, are driven by their need for attention, power, and significance. When they "misbehave," it is a distortion of these needs. The misbehavior is not the problem but rather a symptom of it. When a child is motivated by the need for power, attention, and significance but doesn't know how to achieve these things, they become disheartened. There is a confusing internal conflict between what is naturally felt internally and how the manifestation of those needs is met externally. Seeing problematic behavior as the expression of this confusion has the capacity to transform our view of our kids—to see how similar we are, to rouse compassion, to prioritize helping them (and, indirectly, ourselves) to see clearly, and to assist them in finding their way to an undistorted expression of their needs.

NO BAD KIDS

WHEN MY SON WAS ABOUT four years old, he had a few run-ins with an older child in our building. My son was drawn to older kids and, for the most part, their generosity and gentleness with him surprised me. But this kid was an exception, always a little rougher and gruffer than the others. The momma bear in me pigeonholed this child, labeling him as someone to be careful of, and looked no further. In my mind, he hurt my child and there was nothing else I needed to know. In the time since, however, I have come to understand this child a bit better and to see how his unique combination of temperament, emotional differences, and intelligence culminated in him appearing as a "bad kid." My initial impression of him wasn't even 1 percent of the story.

As always, when I have succumbed to the darkness of over-simplifying and labeling, something happens to show me my ignorance. More recently, my own child has developed some issues—a combination of behavioral, emotional regulation, neurological–sensory, and who knows what else—and I find myself in the unenviable position of wondering if my kid has become *that* kid to any of the other parents. It's a painful point when you alone can see the beautiful depths of your child as well as their sensitivities and limitations, and you fear they could be misunderstood, labeled, or "othered."

Children pick up on these labels and judgments, internalize them, and replay them over the course of their lives. They write their narrative accordingly, casting themselves in the same antagonistic role in each and every scenario. And as a result, they diminish their wholeness, habitually narrowing their character into a predictable course, rather than leaving space for their truly undefinable, expansive, and evolving nature.

Buddha-nature, or basic goodness, holds that each of us is inherently and unwaveringly whole, worthy, and lovable. There may be layers obscuring that goodness at times and for a variety of reasons, but it is always present. A mommysattva can see the basic goodness in her own child as no one else can. She is uniquely poised to help her child realize and maintain a connection with that basic goodness by encouraging them to feel all their feelings and helping them to manage their emotions and work with their own individual challenges. As a result of her modeling and support, a mommysattva's child learns to open and expand into all their emotions as they rise, level off, break, and dissolve.

By creating an environment in which all emotions are welcome, by sharing power with her children, apologizing when she has wronged them, and forgiving easily, the mommysattva renders the emotional landscape much less anxiety- and fear-inducing. Her children can then lean into the spacious, magnificent, and uncertain truths of being human.

CHILDREN ARE BORN
WITH THEIR TEMPERAMENT

EARLY IN MY SON'S ATTEMPTS TO WALK, I captured him on video. He's wearing a white onesie, his right foot still dramatically turned out due to congenital torticollis, and he's pushing a walker toy with a handle to hold on to and adjustable wheels that control the resistance. He has literally just begun but has already grown impatient with himself, with his lack of ease. He is not yet one year old, and he is angry at his limitations.

I think of that video often when I see my son continue to bump up against his limitations. He has a very short fuse, quick to explode when he can't master something on the first try. This isn't laziness or "being difficult." This is the temperament he was born with and it's very, very familiar to me. He will never be an easygoing kid. If I can accept this about him, if I can try not to lament it or fight it or change it, both our lives will be a lot easier.

Rather we can concentrate on the much more productive effort of learning to work with that temperament.

Tending to our children with attention and compassion in full view of the temperament with which they were born preserves their humanity, communicates our deep belief in their basic goodness, and conveys the unconditional love inherent in motherhood. We say with our words and actions, "I love you so much that I will help you to become who you are."

THE ESSENTIAL NATURE OF DISCOMFORT

IT IS HUMAN TO PREFER ease over difficulty. Often, when we experience pain and suffering, we think it's because we're not doing something right. But, as the Buddha taught in his Four Noble Truths, suffering is an inevitable part of life. Resisting that fact is what amplifies our suffering. Accepting it liberates us.

Knowing how to tolerate discomfort in motherhood is key to ultimately allowing our children to be who they are—to walking the fine line between helping them become good citizens who know how to exist in and contribute to society and nurturing their individual personalities, honoring their sovereignty. Everyone superficially acknowledges that motherhood is the hardest job in the world, and yet when certain difficulties arise, our knee-jerk reaction is to diffuse, discharge, and relieve that difficulty ASAP. In our haste to not feel discomfort, however, we miss some of the richest moments of motherhood.

Generosity, discipline, and attention pave the way to understanding how to work with the suffering that is inevitable, how to hold our hearts and minds as we face these challenges alongside our children, and how to come out the other side more connected, wiser, and more confident in the basic goodness we all possess.

RELIEVING THEIR DISCOMFORT

I HAVE SAID, "I wish I could take your pain into my own body" to my son so many times that now, whenever he is injured or upset, he has begun to say, "I wish this had happened to you and not me."

When they are suffering, the pain we feel as mothers cannot be overestimated. Whether a toothache or heartache, we wish to take the throb into our own bodies. This is impossible, of course, but that doesn't stop us from wracking our brains trying to find a way. Sometimes when we do this, we move away from the central problem, the origin of their pain, the dynamic of our own suffering by extension, and distort the situation. Much of this stems from our own intolerance for discomfort, only made more brittle and twitchy by the fact it is being experienced by the person we think of as "our heart walking around outside our bodies."

Of course, we do what we can. We dispense the Tylenol, offer a new toy, soothe with hot chocolate, or just sit and rock with them. We relieve the suffering we can. But how do we tell the difference between a compassionate act of relieving their pain and the act of idiotic compassion that robs them of an experience that could ultimately lead to deeper understanding, tolerance, and resilience?

Oh, were you expecting an answer? Unfortunately, I don't have one. That's because there isn't one answer. This is a moment-by-moment discernment we practice and hone by relating directly to our own pain and fear and intolerance to uncertainty.

Taking each circumstance as it comes, we decide what is needed and take that next step.

HELPING THEM TOLERATE DISCOMFORT

JUST BEFORE MY SON TURNED FOUR, he decided it was time to let go of his binky. This was a scary stage for all of us. Just seeing his nervous system downshift when the "binky–woo-woo solution" was applied ("woo-woo" being his name for his little lamb blanket) had me wondering how I would ever replicate that relief in a way that didn't lead to expensive orthodontal work or long-term cognitive behavioral therapy. We had discussed the decision but left the choice of when up to him.

One morning after waking, he declared, "I am ready to throw out my binky," and pitched it in the garbage can. That whole day, he celebrated his decision, and the moments when he needed some soothing, he stated clearly, "I would usually use my binky–woo-woo, but now I only use the woo-woo."

That night, he lay down in his bed and snuggled his cheek into his woo-woo. Then he looked up at me and said, "Binky?"

That next moment was the emotional equivalent of a ten-car pileup for me: *I knew it! He didn't realize that his decision meant giving it up for good. It would be so much easier to just give him the backup binky. That way he can fall asleep easily and I can go relax. But then we won't be any closer to helping him self-soothe. OMG, he's going to be the only kid crossing the stage to get his high school diploma with a binky in his mouth. Of course, I'm the one making this decision. Where is his dad when I need him?! Oh man, am I willing to ride this rollercoaster?*

What ensued was like watching the five stages of grief unfold at lightning speed. Denial, anger, bargaining, depression—boom, boom, boom, boom. He finally ventured into acceptance, the complex awareness that I trusted him to get through without the binky while staying by his side and sharing in his grief. We both emerged from that night raw and vulnerable but also stronger.

Those moments of discerning whether to relieve their suffering or help them to endure it are many, and there is no rule book. The underlying view that guided me that night was that helping him learn to tolerate discomfort will be one of the most important parts of our relationship and one of the most important things he'll ever learn, something that maintains his sovereignty and helps him grow into someone who is not pathologically driven by the need, to his own detriment, for comfort. Beneath it was a willingness to feel my own pain, a capacity to open to the suffering of my child, and the belief that moving through it together had deep and lasting value.

THEIR URGENCY TO GROW UP

WHEN MY SON WAS THREE YEARS OLD, he couldn't wait to grow up. At any moment he could be found in the apartment carting his step stool around so that he could reach new heights and do more and more on his own. He grew teary whenever something was literally or figuratively out of his reach and expressed his urgency to grow up: "When I'm older I will…" He also detested (and continues to detest) being told what to do, having internalized the false idea that when you grow up you can do whatever you please.

His desire to fast-forward, his frustration and longing for a different emotional state and set of abilities make my heart ache. I know that feeling so well—to wish away a time of your life. To lack the patience and presence to see the sacredness of being right where you are and to having compassion for discontent. Part of me wishes to satisfy his longing for something different while another part of me wishes to convey the preciousness of staying right where he is.

I still don't quite know how to explain the drawbacks of wishing those difficult moments of your life away, and the likelihood of nostalgia for those times wished away. All I know to do in these moments is to hold the space for his restlessness and his dissatisfaction. To attend to his present-moment heart, mind, and body with warmth and openness. To share how I have been there myself, that I understand how painful it is, and at the same time how I have learned that this moment, too, is precious.

OWNING OUR OWN "STUFF"

AN ESSENTIAL COMPONENT of preserving our children's sovereignty is discerning our "stuff" from theirs. Growing up, my dad had a thing about me referring to my mother as "her." I still have no idea why. I assume it came from his own upbringing and, despite the fact that I meant no harm in using this neutral pronoun, you can bet I deployed it when I wanted to push buttons. The point is that he confused his own stuff with mine in a way that only increased our collective confusion.

I often see this tendency in myself. For example, whenever my son slams the door—whether this is done intentionally or as a result of a vacuum created by an open window—my brain shuts down and all rational thought ceases. Something is triggered, and it is as if he has violated some unwritten rule of parent–child interaction. The first one hundred times it happened I found myself becoming indignant, bursting into his room to reprimand him. Eventually, I started to see slammed doors as my own ancient association with disrespect, lack of parental "control," and ruptured communication. Slammed doors terrified me. What helped me recognize this as my own baggage was looking into his tearful, fearful eyes as I unleashed an energy that had nothing to do with him.

The Buddhist view of meditation in everyday life is that each experience, no matter how seemingly small, presents us with an opportunity to either wake up or to go further to sleep; to recognize the nature of reality—what is actually happening in a given moment—or solidify our confusion in a way that obscures our natural state of enlightenment. Our children unwittingly unearth our ancient history so that we are confronted with it in powerful ways. In the heat of the moment it is easy to succumb to the shutdown of blame, aggression, and the illusion of separateness. With attention and practice, it becomes more and more possible to catch ourselves and transform that confusion into wisdom and compassion.

APOLOGIZING

WHEN I HAVE DONE SOMETHING WRONG, when I have not respected my son's sovereignty, when I have betrayed his trust or failed to keep my word, I own it. I take responsibility and apologize specifically for what I did. What I have learned is that it is a huge relief to apologize to my kid.

Apologizing can feel fraught. How do we maintain our position as "the one who knows better" while also admitting wrongdoing? Doesn't that upset the balance of power, potentially undermining our attempts to guide him or her later on?

Saying "I'm sorry"—authentically, with humility—to our kids is yet another way in which we work with things as they are. We acknowledge that something has transpired we both know was wrong. It speaks what could easily remain unspoken. It is courageous and radical.

Taking responsibility for our wrongdoings reinforces the humanity of our kids. It communicates that they are whole beings worthy of respect and that receiving an apology is not just adult territory. As a result, they learn to take responsibility for themselves, their mistakes, and the ways in which they may harm others.

FORGIVING EASILY

AT TIMES, OUR KIDS will really hurt or disappoint us. They will make our lives uncomfortable. They will show us aspects of themselves we didn't want to see and aspects of ourselves we never anticipated. In those moments of collapse, how we respond determines how our children learn to work with hurt and disappointment.

Our ability to acknowledge and let go of these moments, to communicate the difference between the person and the action, determines not just how we move forward in the short term but how our relationship—and our child's self-image—ripens over time. When we withhold affection, withdraw our warmth, wield the emotional hangover of an incident against our children in the aftermath, we introduce doubt about their basic goodness and about our unspoken promise to ride the rollercoaster together. We may do this because it was how we were raised, but holding a grudge is not discipline. It's inhumane, an enactment of our own confusion, our wish for control, and our fear of groundlessness.

How quickly and authentically we forgive speaks volumes. Even if a behavior is bad, true forgiveness reinforces our children's Buddha-nature, humanity, and sovereignty. True forgiveness teaches them to let go of what has already happened and come into the present moment. To stop living in the past. To release grudges. To let go of settling the score.

We will not always get this right, but getting it right is not the point. And the good news is that there will be plenty of opportunities to practice, many opportunities to forgive one another.

BITTERSWEET CELEBRATIONS

TOSSING BASKETBALLS UNDERHAND at the playground one day, my son reached a familiar breaking point when he bumped up against his limitations. Never mind the fact that the backboards are NBA regulation height and he is all of three feet tall. His irritable perfectionism requires him to overcome such odds, immediately and consistently. When he is so painfully hard on himself, my heartbreak often manifests as frustration at his frustration, and this leads to so much hurt. This interaction was no exception and he registered a need to be separate from me in order to reset.

"Mommy, can I please go over there by myself?" he asked me when we both were about to explode. The swell of emotions I felt in that moment was indescribable: proud of his self-awareness and his ability to verbalize his needs, fear and worry at the thought of him struggling like this throughout his life, dismay at how I had contributed to this moment of confusion, disappointment that the resolution to this problem would not in fact come from me. So proud and so heartbroken.

The word "bittersweet" fails to capture the collision of emotions we mothers experience as our babies grow into themselves. The bliss of watching them achieve new milestones is matched only by the simultaneous agony of knowing that with each new step (literal and figurative) they move farther away from us.

ALL EMOTIONS ARE WELCOME

WHEN I WAS EIGHT MONTHS PREGNANT, my partner and I went to see Pixar's *Inside Out*. Early on in the movie, the protagonist Riley's emotions are ruled by Joy. Joy runs the show and manages the "negative" contributions of disgust, anger, fear, and, particularly, sadness. As the movie progresses and Riley faces the pain of moving to a new city and going to an unfamiliar school, her one-note core memories are replaced by more complex ones that are tinged by multiple emotions simultaneously. She discovers that it is her capacity to welcome the full spectrum of her emotional experience that gives her access to unfathomable richness in life.

When we consider how many of our personal and global problems stem from our intolerance of those "negative emotions"—our inability to assertively and compassionately face conflict, our need to fast-forward through sadness or loneliness or grief, our failure to face head-on how our pleasure seeking now contributes to pain later—the need to welcome all our emotions starts to come into focus.

It is a gift to help our children welcome all their emotions. To model this, discuss it, guide them to open to the full range. Imagine what life would be like if we knew deep in our bones that all emotions were welcome and inherently good. That our sadness and rage were as important to feel and make space for as our joy and contentment.

MASCULINE AND FEMININE

IN COLLEGE, MY WOMEN'S STUDIES PROFESSOR pointed out how obsessed we are with the sex of a new baby, usually long before it's born, as if that were the most important piece of information. Examples of gendered treatment begin just as early—hospital nursery signs reading "I'm a boy" or "It's a girl," suggesting different levels of personal agency. Once they have begun, they never let up. My son was admonished early on by others for crying, using a pacifier, and wearing nail polish. Some mothers fear their daughters might be bossy, mean, or, as I heard in one particularly disturbing comment from a mom group attendee, "crazy or a bitch" (the child was six months old).

Our overemphasis on gender reveals our assumption that it dictates everything we need to know about an individual. What his or her or their personality, preferences, and path are likely to be. What we often fail to appreciate is that our children naturally possess both masculine and feminine qualities that are not dictated by their chromosomes. They are born this way, and it is up to us above all others to help them maintain this wholeness, knowing full well that our culture will try its best to beat it out of them.

One of many ways we preserve the sovereignty of our children is to respect and nurture the masculine and feminine energies in all of them. To do this we must investigate our own internalized sexism, subscription to heteronormativity, and attachment to gender norms. From the very beginning, seeing that convenient gendered portrayals of male and female characters—the muscle-bound superheroes, the eye-batting damsels in distress—cause harm and offer no benefit other than conformity is invaluable. Processing these things with our children allows them to discover themselves, for themselves. Treating children as dynamic bundles of idiosyncratic masculine and feminine qualities contributes to a society of more complex and even more thoughtful humans with tolerance for all displays of inner and outer variations. In other words, it helps children develop their innate compassion and imaginations.

When my son turned two, he received four cars and two trucks. His favorite toy at the time? A blue gingham-checked baby stroller, which I purchased for him after he kept stealing baby strollers from girls in the park. He had no use for cars and trucks at that time. A more apt gift for his second birthday might therefore have been a baby to push in the stroller. But that did not happen. Three years on and among his favorite toys are—wait for it—cars and trucks. I did my very best to go with the cars phase without prejudice.

Our embodiment of masculine and feminine qualities determines basically everything: close relationships, feeling and showing of emotion, comfort with vulnerability, confidence in our abilities, et cetera. What we perceive as masculine and feminine qualities in our current societal and psychological norms are often significantly distorted from their pure origins. The essence of the masculine is active and dynamic; the essence of the feminine is spacious and still. In Tantric Buddhism, this balance of moving through space and being space is the fundamental insight on which the entire path hinges. How we welcome the masculine and feminine in our sons and daughters has everything to do with how we relate to these fundamental energies in ourselves.

RESPECTING OUR KIDS' BODIES

OUR BODIES ARE THE CONTROL CENTERS from which we experience everything. Our kids are born with a relatively uncomplicated relationship with their bodies. Inevitably, that grows more complex with age, changes, and interactions with people and situations. It is our role as mommysattvas to help them navigate this evolution with a sense of confidence and agency.

When they are very young, our children's bodies are a province that we govern. We are in near complete control when they lack the capacity to feed themselves, go to the bathroom, move from place to place. But that changes, sometimes gradually, other times seemingly overnight. Our role then is to perceive those changes, respond to them in real time, and adapt our thoughts and behavior accordingly.

What can seem harmless—tickling your child against their will, forcing them to hug relatives, picking them up and bringing them where you want them to be when they don't follow your orders, staking dessert on finishing their vegetables—can confuse a child about who is in charge of their bodies. It can simultaneously say "yours" and "not yours." Preserving the sovereignty of their bodies communicates that their bodies are no one's but their own, that they are the authorities who know best what is arising inside of them as they learn exactly how best to care for themselves.

The body can be a forgotten element of spiritual practice. Wording it "mindfulness" suggests that spiritual practice occurs in the mental space, not venturing below the neck, not concerned with the mundanity of physical needs, desires, appetites, sensations. This is different from the body being a "temple" that is to be revered—instead, it is rather ordinary and at the same time precious.

The first of the mind-training slogans, "First, train in the preliminaries," reminds us of the preciousness of a human birth. How being born into these exquisitely complex bodies gives us access to the sensations with which we experience the world and allows us to practice the *dharma*, to learn to wake up to the nature of reality. That this awakening is not relegated to the mind but rather to the whole being. Keeping this in mind, we foster our children's mind–body integration.

FOOD

ONE OF THE VERY FIRST WAYS our children establish their autonomy is through their relationship with food. Children are naturally connected with their body's sensations of hunger and fullness, and there is no additional "noise" yet to distort their precise reactions to these sensations. When a child is hungry, she cries for food. When she is satisfied, she turns away from the breast or bottle, purses her lips to refuse another spoonful of sweet potato. As they get older, tastes and preferences continue to change. They also become vulnerable to the influence of siblings, friends, and adults. Kids may go through phases of preferences and aversions, and our reactions to these shifts and changes are key to how they come through them. Our job as mommysattvas is to respect and nurture our children so that they maintain the connection with their bodies and this healthy relationship with food.

Our collective anxiety about health, growth, development, and our children's bodies can lead us to intervene in ways that disturb their natural ability to self-regulate. Though the intentions are good, the impact may be that children learn not to trust what their bodies are telling them. We unwittingly pass to our children the anxieties that we developed or received from those caring for us. And when we engage in power struggles over food—rather than supporting our children's natural capacity for regulation—we may unintentionally end up further distorting their relationship with food and by extension their bodies.

On the other hand, if we model trust in our bodies—in their innate intelligence and capacity for adaptation—our children will learn to balance inside information with outside information as they grow and develop.

Two child-feeding models, Ellyn Satter's Division of Responsibility (DOR) and Evelyn Tribole and Elyse Resch's Intuitive Eating, offer mothers a framework to remove our anxiety and support our children's natural healthy relationship with food. In DOR, parents decide what is served as well as when and where. Children get to decide whether they eat and how much. Intuitive Eating comprises ten principles that place allegiance with the body's sensations and centers satisfaction, which only the individual can sense and respond to.

These approaches create a "container" in which a healthy relationship with food is nurtured and sustained. In Buddhist philosophy, the container principle says that the environment in which something happens influences what happens and what happens influences the environment. The environment created by DOR and Intuitive Eating conveys that kids are responsible for receiving and responding to signals from their own bodies and that the parent will continue to supply a variety of foods, to support their ability to choose, and to not create a situation in which children are rebelling, resisting, sneaking, hiding, and behaving in ways that conflict with their own bodies.

Similar to Buddhist philosophy, DOR and Intuitive Eating are based on a deep and abiding trust in the individual's perception of and judgment in caring for their own bodies. These two models acknowledge that when free from judgment, shame, and arbitrary restrictions, our children can naturally maintain their connection with their bodies and nurture a peaceful relationship with food for the duration of their lives.

CHILDREN AND BODY IMAGE

OUR CHILDREN EXPRESS THEIR BUDDHA-NATURE with their whole selves. There is no separation between mind and heart and body. Mommy Sangha member Emma describes how her daughter registers joy with her whole body:

> She doesn't attempt to filter it with her mind or experience first. It's just a physical explosion. Her eyes sparkle; she raises on tippy toes and exclaims. It's instant. Her hair almost springs up too, like how a dog wriggles and their ears perk up when happy. When she runs toward something you can see the intent in her whole body. A fullness and force of attention.

This natural capacity to feel and express extends to their suffering as well as their joy. My son is gradually developing the language to describe what is happening in his body as he starts to "freak out." As his frustration with his limitations rises, he can consciously feel the sensation of his throat closing, his eyes burning, the grimace taking shape on his face. This real-time awareness allows him to work with his nervous system, interrupting the momentum of the breakdown to consciously soothe with a breath, a hug, or through tears.

As mommysattvas, especially if fueled by our own positive relationship with our bodies, we have the capacity to nourish our children's body image so that they trust their bodies, receive the body's messages and respond to them in real time, inhabit their bodies fully to live their lives sensually, fully. Because children know no separation between body and mind, we can help them maintain that connection, so that they remain fully aware of the basic goodness of their bodies—of every body—and so that they can nurture this long-term relationship that provides them with the ground for their own spiritual practice.

MOTHERS AS
SOCIAL JUSTICE

MY SON WAS BORN TOWARD the end of President Obama's second term. The political climate was shifting in radical and destabilizing ways. It became clear as the 2016 election neared that whomever we chose, it would make history. I took my son with me to vote, affixed my "I voted" sticker to his tiny jacket after casting my ballot for the first female president of the United States, and hosted an election party against my better maternal judgment, knowing it would cost me precious sleep. Just across town at the Javits Center, the party wasn't happening for Hillary Clinton.

The election hit me in a peculiar way as a mother. How would it impact this child to grow up in a country run by someone who bragged about grabbing women "by the pussy"? Who summarized immigration from Mexico as "They're bringing drugs; they're bringing crime. They're rapists and some, I assume, are good people..."? Who would go on to conduct unintelligible COVID briefings and suggest, "Suppose that we hit the body with a tremendous—whether it's ultraviolet or just very powerful—light," and ask, "Is there a way we can do something like [using disinfectant] by injection inside or almost a cleaning?"?

Had I lived through this scenario and not been a mother, I would have fallen into a depression, curled up in a ball, resigned to the perversity of it all. Instead, motivated by love and rage, I found new motivation to get involved with politics and social justice movements. I donated and marched and joined organizations that fight for equity for all. I delved into resources for how to raise a strong, sensitive, feminist, anti-racist boy, sought out ways to work with his fierce temperament so that he learned how to mobilize for good, and often wove in discussions of how to be a decent human that greets the world and all its inhabitants with compassion and empathy.

I know you love your child(ren) more than anything. I know that you want to do right by them while also having a sense of stability and meaning for yourself. I assume that you have at least begun to see that there is no real separation between "you" and "me" or between any two human beings, no matter their location, background, experience—that we all want the same things: safety, inclusion, respect, visibility, significance, and meaning.

As our children grow and change, our awareness of them— their suffering, their joy, their deep humanity—expands. At the same time, our awareness of and compassion for all beings must also expand. In one way or another, all mothers engage with the social, political, environmental, and educational systems that can nourish or poison our children. Though we may wish to withdraw and pull back from the world, giving up our privacy as mommy-sattvas means we are constantly opening to the world and its needs.

Mothers are inherently on the frontlines of global social justice movements if only because of how they prepare children to interact with the world and its inhabitants. So much of how every individual exists in the world—how they impact one another, what they prioritize, who they benefit, who they harm, how they work with their own confusion—is influenced by that primary relationship with their mothers.

The Buddhist path is inextricable from righteous activism. In committing to work with our minds through the lens of the *dharma*—the truth—we must challenge our confusion, fear, selfishness, and ignorance. The Noble Eightfold Path—the path to liberation that acknowledges the truth of suffering and our resistance to it—includes right view, right intention, right speech, right action, right livelihood, right effort, right mindfulness, and right concentration. As nondualistic as Buddhist philosophy is— that is, black and white, good and bad do not inherently exist— there are certain inalienable truths: all beings are basically good and deserve the same compassion, kindness, safety, health, and peace, both inner and outer.

In other words, the mommysattva is spiritually incapable of resting in blissful ignorance.

Mothers have long been at the forefront of social justice movements made necessary by the tragic and needless deaths of their children. Mothers have mobilized against bullying, unsafe work conditions, drunk driving, gun violence, the disproportionate victimization of Black and brown bodies, and violence against women, girls, and gay, bisexual, and transgender individuals.

I grew up in the 1980s when Mothers Against Drunk Driving came into existence. The movement was born after Cari Lightner was struck and killed by a repeat drunk driver. Her mother, Candace, carrying a picture of her daughter everywhere, fought to raise awareness and spark action against driving under the influence of alcohol or drugs. Even as a child, the neat encapsulation of a mother's rage in this movement's acronym was clear to me. MADD caught our attention not only because many of its leaders were SAHMs, suddenly and vocally front and center in unexpected leadership roles, but also because of the force of their anger, their cries of pain, their fierce action and coordination and demands.

In the early 1990s, after her son was stricken with a chronic health condition, housewife-turned-activist Lois Gibbs began the Love Canal Homeowners Association to stop toxic chemicals from being dumped in her New York town. Moms Demand Action was created in the wake of the Sandy Hook massacre in 2012. After Florida teenager Trayvon Martin's murderer, George Zimmerman, was acquitted, Sybrina Fulton and other members of Mothers of the Movement spoke at the 2016 Democratic National Convention, made several media appearances, including one with Beyoncé at the Video Music Awards that year, and were a significant presence in the 2017 Women's March. Before the mostly white "Wall of Moms" locked arms in Portland, Oregon, in 2020 to form a barrier between protesters in the Black Lives Matter movement and armed federal agents, the mostly Black "Army of Moms" set up shop on the streets of Englewood, Chicago, to prevent more senseless shootings of Black bodies. And after video footage revealed that in his final moments George Floyd had called out for his mother, fellow mother Rachel Costa's protest sign went viral. It stated simply, "All mothers were summoned when George Floyd called out for his momma." When someone's child—anyone's child—is harmed, the mother's warriorship is invoked instinctively, involuntarily.

When I was seven months pregnant, I witnessed a near accident at an intersection by Memorial Sloan Kettering Cancer Center. A woman fresh out of chemotherapy hazily crossed the street—she had the right of way—when an exhausted shift worker heading home turned into the intersection, nearly striking her. When he slammed on the brakes, time stopped. Everyone in the vicinity froze, their collective consciousness still playing out what could have happened. I broke out of my paralysis and walked into the center of the intersection, took the trembling woman by the arm and accompanied her to the curb where she broke down, and was soon joined by the driver who had pulled over to come to her aid.

A year later, as I pushed the stroller toward the same corner, a nearly identical almost-accident unfolded. This time, tethered to my child, it was clear that it would not be my body entering the intersection. I had to leave that to someone else. What I could do was to open my heart to the individuals involved, the pedestrian, the driver, those capable of taking bodily action, and all those witnesses suddenly very aware of their mortality. In that moment, I became aware of how my capacity for righteous action had changed and would continue to change. And I realized the opportunity to reframe how to be present in a moment and a movement.

As mommysattvas, we may need to challenge our own definition of what it means to take action for justice. At times activism is outward—marching, keening her truth, crying for justice, lobbying for just and impartial laws. Often her action is inner, more subtle, perhaps even invisible. The mommysattva understands that this flexibility is essential to working with things as they are, to addressing the causes of change at home and, when possible, to contributing to change on a larger scale. She challenges her own vulnerability to performative activism in which there must be witnesses of her good deeds, competitive wokeness in which she engages in a contest for righteousness, and self-protective withdrawal where she distances herself from her ignorance and the discomfort inherent in confronting it directly. She continually works with her own mind, assimilating the various pieces of the puzzle, clearly seeing the direct lines between the individuals in her charge and the grander scheme of how beings relate to one another.

With her body and heart–mind as her weapons, the mommysattva is the protector and action taker when the safety of her children—the safety of all children—is threatened.

RAISING FEMINISTS

WHEN I WENT OFF TO COLLEGE, I'd not yet identified as a feminist. Growing up, it was considered a sort of F-word, and few were willing to assume that mantle for fear of being called a "man-hater." Once I took a Women's Studies 101 class, I was forever changed. One quote that cut through all the propaganda about what the F-word actually means was "Feminism is the radical notion that women are people." (I've since learned that this often-misattributed quote was actually coined by writer, editor, and Brooklyn native Marie Shear.) Now I wonder how anyone could not consider themselves feminist (though I do realize that this word has come to mean a feminism only beneficial to white women, and that therefore it is essential to be a proponent of intersectional feminism).

As evidenced by titles such as bell hooks' *Feminism Is for Everybody: Passionate Politics*, the argument has been made that feminism is not just for women. Regardless of religious or political views, how can one seriously assert that women are not deserving of equal opportunities and equal wages for equal work, of influence on policies that impact the female body, of safety from violence? Contemplating the dharma—again, often translated as "the truth"—is it not clear both that we are equal and that brutal inequities persist? Can we not see how a rising tide lifts all boats? The issue is huge and overwhelming, but perhaps we could begin by looking at the gender politics in our own homes.

The early influence of sexism on our children's consciousness is startling: "gender reveal" parties before a child is even born; boys gifted toy guns, girls gifted dollies; sports divisions; gender-targeted marketing and advertising. There is a direct effect when a boy grows up seeing his mother cover all domestic tasks while his father puts up his feet. When anger is tolerated in males but not in females. When tears are tended to in girls and shamed in boys. These seemingly minor issues all add up, contributing to and upholding systems of gender-based discrimination. Our interruption of them has the potential to change underlying beliefs—our own and those burgeoning beliefs of our children.

As mothers, we have the power to rebalance our children's perspectives on themselves as boys or girls or nonbinary or any other gender expression and on their gender-based expectations. We can point out where our culture pigeonholes them, challenge how this limited programming detracts from our wholeness, and encourage and accompany our kids in inhabiting and embracing their own masculinity and femininity as well as that of others.

Noticing, calling out (or calling in—see page 232), and interrupting sexist practices in our own homes has the capacity to normalize feminism, to help our children to see the connections between their subtle beliefs about gender and the pain and harm that often falls on women because of those beliefs.

VIOLENCE AGAINST WOMEN
IS A MEN'S ISSUE

ONE OF THE THREE MARKS OF EXISTENCE is no self (or egolessness): the interdependence of all beings and the absence of any real separation between us. The thoughts we think, the words we speak, the actions we take, they do not affect a single individual; rather, they affect all of us. Everything we put into the world influences the collective experience. The question is, will our experiences help us to wake up or go further to sleep? How we raise our children to embrace their whole selves and care for one another is the answer to this question.

From the moment I learned the sex of my child, I have been determined to raise a feminist who neither directly participates in nor indirectly fosters sexism and violence against women and girls. To that end, I have always tried to drive home to my son the importance of listening to and respecting everyone's wishes for how their bodies are treated. If someone does not want a hug, I tell him to love them from afar. If someone he's playing rough with suddenly wishes to downshift, I tell him to listen to their words, pay attention to their body language, and do what is necessary to honor their wishes.

Jackson Katz, an American educator and the first man to minor in Women's Studies at the University of Massachusetts Amherst, has worked with national sports teams and the US military to educate men to take responsibility for ending violence against women. He has stated that "violence against women is a men's issue" and that "it is anti-male to not be doing this work."

Paul Lacerte, an Indigenous Canadian man—and father of a daughter—founded the Moose Hide Campaign to help end violence toward women and children. The organization supports and amplifies the voices of survivors, supports and holds accountable other men, and teaches young boys what it really means to love, respect, and protect one another.

Traditionally, the paradigm has been to focus on the victim and perpetrator of a violent incident, falsely reducing the incident to an interaction between two separate people—separate from one another and separate from the rest of us. This binary is a fallacy that does nothing to address the systemic roots of violence against women and the collective responsibility we have in protecting our fellow humans.

Long before men commit violence against women, boys are encouraged to distance themselves from what is considered feminine—crying, being affectionate, voicing their emotions. Not only are boys pushed to disavow their softer side, they are also expected to power over the feminine. This is how relationships between boys and girls become conquests of the former over the latter. The implicit message to boys is "Exorcise the feminine in yourself and then obliterate the feminine outside of you." It is not hard to understand how this occurs on countless individual levels only to culminate in a system that affects all of us.

Girls, on the other hand, bombarded by messages about how they should look, feel, think, and act, seem to have little choice but to internalize sexist and misogynistic themes. They then weaponize those themes against themselves and other females. They learn to satisfy the male gaze, to not rock the boat, to do it all, and to judge harshly anyone not falling in line. However, if skillfully presented with the whole story—that we all possess masculine and feminine qualities and that it is this wholeness that allows us to find balance and to enact right action—girls can draw their own conclusions and realize their truth.

Gender-based violence always stems from some instance of the perpetrator believing he is independent of his victim. That hurting another body is different from hurting one's own body or hurting all bodies. In the wake of violence against female bodies, there is the inevitable plea to imagine if the victim were your mother, your sister, your daughter—as if the only way to understand such violence is in a personal capacity. One should not need a sister, mother, or daughter to abhor violence against women, to understand that it is at endemic proportions, to see how it touches and affects all facets of society, and to want it to end.

RAISING ANTI-RACIST KIDS

THE FOLLOWING IS WRITTEN SPECIFICALLY for other white moms.

As inhabitants of a country built on the theft of land and genocide of Indigenous people and subsequent chattel slavery, the white population in the United States has inherited the karma of racism that has yet to be adequately and appropriately acknowledged, atoned for, and reconciled. Though our own families may not have personally perpetrated the original offenses, we inevitably participate in and benefit from the present-day systems that uphold racism (or "white-body supremacy," a term used by Resmaa Menakem in his book *My Grandmother's Hands: Racialized Trauma and the Pathway to Mending Our Hearts and Bodies*). We may not have been explicitly taught in school to be anti-racist, but that does not exempt us from educating ourselves now. The history of chattel slavery in our country, fictional and nonfictional accounts written by people of color, and scientific data demonstrating evidence of systemic racism are all widely available. It is our responsibility to see what we might rather not see. Once it is seen, it cannot be unseen.

From a Buddhist viewpoint, the origins of these atrocities and their present-day manifestations stem from a profound confusion about our interdependence—how we are all connected and how there is no true separation between one person and another. In the words of Audre Lorde, "I am not free while any woman is unfree, even when her shackles are very different from my own. And I am not free as long as one person of Color remains chained. Nor is any one of you."

It is no longer enough to be "not racist"—in truth, it never was. As mommysattvas, we must take personal responsibility to learn and understand how systemic racism arose and endured in our country and to directly oppose it. (This is also an issue in other countries, but the US and other colonizing countries have their own very particular and disturbing relationship with racism.) There is no easy way to do this. There are no shortcuts to recognizing these truths, though that doesn't stop us from trying to find them: apologizing just to appease, quickly switching into problem-solving mode, preferring to do something other than sit with the uncomfortable knowledge of our complicity, disavowing our participation in the systems that cause harm, perseverating on our intent when our impact was harmful, claiming that we, too, have suffered traumas such as poverty (even if we still benefit from white privilege) or reverse racism (which simply does not exist—if you don't agree, call me. We'll talk).

The capacity for anti-racism work is directly tied to our ability and willingness to look truthfully at ourselves, our loved ones, and our communities. All the anti-racism resources I've read inevitably speak to the need to experience discomfort (in our hearts and in our bodies) and to move toward what scares us. As Rhonda V. Magee, author of *The Inner Work of Racial Justice: Healing Ourselves and Transforming Our Communities Through Mindfulness*, puts it:

> The process of becoming mindful can assist us in knowing ourselves, being more familiar with the habits of our minds and our own emotional reactivity—the anger, confusion, numbness, and outrage that arise when we see racism. It helps us become more self-compassionate and, thus, minimizes the drama of encountering racism.

Meditation provides us with the tools we need to do anti-racism work: the capacity to sit with our discomfort and look deeply and honestly at ourselves; the ability to recognize how painful it is to feel the realities of racism and how readily we would like to change that experience through seemingly productive or even baldly unproductive ways.

Once we commit to becoming anti-racist, it can be daunting to know where to begin. As moms, we are already short on time and other limited resources. It's great if we can donate to anti-racist causes, volunteer our time, or use our bodies to demonstrate in support of necessary causes such as the Black Lives Matter movement, but the most potent anti-racist work we can do is to raise anti-racist kids. Mothers who are Black, Indigenous, and people of color do not have a choice over whether or not to have difficult conversations with their children about race—why people treat them differently, how to pacify white people so as not to appear threatening, how to not get shot by the police. Until all mothers do not have to warn their children about the products of racism, all mothers need to have these conversations.

The conversation won't be distinct or isolated. More likely, it will be a conversation we begin and then allow to unfold in installments over time. It might be pointing out how the villain in a story "happens to be" a person of color. It might be encouraging our kids to notice what their doctors, dentists, teachers, coaches, and friends look like and don't look like. It might be encouraging our kids to seek out relationships with people of different backgrounds—not expecting them to educate us about racism, but to learn who they are, what they love and fear, to move through the world with them.

FAT LIBERATION

OUR CULTURE IMPLICITLY AND EXPLICITLY dictates that only thin bodies are worthy bodies, well bodies, bodies deserving of love and respect. Even within the scientific and medical communities, this belief is rampant. As a nutrition grad student, I was trained that ob*sity is at the root of countless chronic diseases, enormous health care costs, and general moral disintegration. Yet the farther I have moved from that traditional training and the deeper I have gotten into the actual scientific research—including that on social determinants of health—the more I have been able to decouple my own confusion from the reality as shown by the data.

Some facts:

> Body weight is determined mostly by factors out of our individual control, such as genetics.
> Being in a larger body does not cause disease or decrease lifespan.

> The BMI is racist and does not accurately measure health.
> Losing weight does not implicitly improve health.
> Dieting is the strongest predictor of long-term weight gain.
> Weight loss is not sustainable for 95 percent of the population.
> The few who are able to maintain weight loss often meet the criteria for disordered eating.

Our confusion around this topic has been subtly (or not so subtly) used to justify bias against people in larger bodies. We are programmed by a sick culture to believe that fat is bad and that people in larger bodies not only possess negative personality characteristics, like laziness and gluttony, but also are actually in full control of their weight and so essentially choose to be fat. What we fail to acknowledge is that the true link between fat and disease is our collective bias against fat bodies. Like any other form of discrimination on the basis of a single oversimplified and misunderstood factor, bias against fat bodies kills.

All of us are touched by fat bias, whether it's the fears that bubble up when our toddler or teenager grows out instead of up, our battle with our own bodies as we age and move through various stages of life, or our statements and judgments about people in larger bodies, known and unknown to us personally.

Fat bias distorts our natural ability to self-regulate eating and movement and makes worthiness contingent upon thinness. It prevents us from looking beyond superficial judgments to see the humans that are harmed by it—humans who desire the same safety, health, happiness, and ease as any of us do. And all humans, not in spite of their differences but in full view and appreciation of them, deserve the same rights and access. This is not something on which we can agree to disagree.

We may not be at fault for the fat bias we internalized as the result of our cultural programming. We are, however, responsible for whether or not we confront this baseless prejudice and perpetuate it within our families and with our children. Maybe not our fault, but our responsibility.

DEFENDING DIFFERENCE

IN OUR APARTMENT COMPLEX'S COURTYARD, roving packs of children of all different ages and backgrounds play, ride scooters, kick soccer balls, make discoveries, fight and make up. It is a separate and semi-protected world within the world of New York City. The unifying features of all these kids is their shared address and their need for connection. During the pandemic, when everyone was sheltering in place and relatively cut off from the outside world, the courtyard offered fresh air and a parcel of space for our rambunctious children.

One day, as a socially distanced birthday party wound down and restless, masked kids ran from one corner of the courtyard to another, one of our neighbors, a beautiful and sweet boy who has Tourette's Syndrome, began to experience one of his tics, uttering an unusual string of words at a high pitch. The boys he was playing with, made uncomfortable by this unexplained difference, told him to stop, joked about what he was saying, and "othered" him. Ultimately, our neighbor left the garden and retreated to the safety and familiarity of his apartment.

Another neighbor of ours, a scientist and fiercely protective empath familiar with being "othered," having witnessed the incident, explained to the boys what they had observed. She told them that our neighbor's tic is a difference he has no control over and that they should not make fun of him. The boys were taken aback. They were confronted with their own ignorance in no uncertain terms, which now put them in the precarious position of either opening up to or shutting down this new perspective.

The moment was a transmission of sorts, a transfer of wisdom that empowers an individual to achieve a higher level of understanding. Such a transmission is an offering from one who has realized an insight to another who possesses that insight but has not yet accessed it. How do we come to know what we do not already know unless someone or something shows us? Such a moment of transmission, if regarded as such, can transcend the shame and embarrassment arising out of ignorance and offer us a new form of awareness.

From an evolutionary standpoint, genetic differences strengthen a population, making them less vulnerable to threats. Why should sociological differences be any different than biological ones? Each of us possesses some way in which we are different. Some peculiarity, preference, or identifying feature. Our differences, or more accurately how they are held and responded to by ourselves and others, can either threaten or satisfy our universal need for belonging and significance. When our differences are accepted as part of the whole person—not what matters most by any means, not problems to be fixed or exorcised—we thrive, as individuals and as communities. When our differences are used as the rationale for exclusion, we all pay the price.

DIFFERENTLY ABLED

AS A CHILD, I WAS VERY CONSCIOUS of two family members who were differently abled. I had a blind cousin, to whom I wrote letters so that I could learn about his life, what he liked to do, what was important to him. Stevie was a confident guy; he had always lived with his disability and had access to the support systems that helped him live a fulfilling and productive life. My maternal grandfather, on the other hand, suffered from a degenerative neuromuscular disease that changed him from an energetic NYPD narcotics officer into a quadriplegic. Unlike Stevie, my Pop Pop felt so much shame at the dissolution of his body and abilities that he became depressed and homebound and withdrew completely from society. The awareness of these two individuals and their different relationships with their disabilities made me sensitive to others with disabilities. I saw how people looked past those in wheelchairs or pretended not to see someone walking with a cane. So I made sure to see them. To look them in the eye. To make sure they knew that I knew they were there.

Growing up in New York City, my son has been exposed to people from every imaginable walk of life—age, race, socioeconomic class, gender identity, ability, and beyond. Because children notice everything and are naturally curious, he is always asking questions, which has given us plenty of opportunities to talk about the different experiences people have in part because of their differently abled bodies. As a result, he has developed an appreciation of difference. He asks his pediatrician about her limb difference, spots the special taxis in town that can accommodate wheelchairs, repeats to me the purpose of the adaptive crosswalks that speak directions for the visually impaired, and runs his fingers over the braille floor numbers in our elevator.

Raising our children to see everyone, to include everyone, to offer everyone the same kindness and compassion as anyone else, connects them with their basic intelligence. It confirms for them how we all wish for the same things: to be appreciated, seen and heard, included, safe, and significant. To do this, we might have to look at our own limitations, what causes us to shut down or even just feel mildly uncomfortable. To confront what we might rather not. Meditation and the underlying view of Buddhism provide us with the tools to do this: to rouse the courage necessary to move toward the very things we naturally shy away from.

DESTIGMATIZING MENTAL ILLNESS

NOT ALL DISABILITIES ARE VISIBLE. Many of us—myself included—struggle with mental illnesses that significantly influence our lives as individuals, mothers, and partners. Mental illness is often poorly understood, not only due to its invisibility but also to the stigma attached to it. This stigma can include feelings of personal responsibility and failure, defectiveness, and danger. Whether we ourselves struggle with mental illness or are somehow touched by the mental illness of another, the topic can show us our edge.

Even the words "mental illness" might cause you to stiffen, to think that it happens to "other people," to wish to gloss over it and move on to more savory topics. But it is very likely that we or our children will experience some form of mental illness over the course of our lives. The term "mental illness" refers to a huge array of cognitive, emotional, and developmental disorders that affect mental functioning. Some are more commonplace, like depression, anxiety, eating disorders, post-traumatic stress disorder, obsessive-compulsive disorder, addiction, autism spectrum disorder, and attention deficit–hyperactivity disorder. Others feel more difficult to consider: bipolar disorder, borderline personality disorder, schizophrenia, psychosis, dissociative disorders, and more.

Living with mental illness is hard enough without the shame and secrecy that often accompany it. Stigma causes people to hide their mental illness, ignoring its specific needs, not getting the support they desperately need from therapists, psychiatrists, and other clinicians, not to mention friends and family members. When mental illness is not addressed directly, life gets distorted. Substance abuse, relationship and work difficulties, and a legacy of trauma are unfortunate and very common effects of unaddressed mental illness. These issues then appear to be the problem when in fact they are just symptoms. They, too, are handed down, creating a snowball effect in which layers of harmful and distracting symptoms are compounded, continually obscuring the original, central issue. Breaking this cycle is exceedingly difficult and cannot be done in a vacuum.

If we were able to remove the stigma attached to mental illness—regarding it both as a component of what makes an individual unique and as part of their experience they must actively work with over the course of their lives—people would be freer to get the help they need, to share their experience, to work openly and directly with their challenges. Removing the stigma attached to mental illness requires us to work with our own discomfort, biases, and beliefs in a way that is kind, honest, and compassionate. To take an unflinching look at ourselves, our family members, the people in our communities, perhaps our own children. To be willing to feel uncomfortable in the interest of working with things as they are.

CALLING IN

SOMETIMES WE DO HARM. It may not be intentional, but nevertheless our impact is hurtful. When we do harm, we may be called out, which highlights the fact that we have done something oppressive. Calling out is a way of holding us accountable and responsible for our words and actions; it can be an opportunity to see ourselves and our capacity to injure others, however unintentionally. But it may have unanticipated consequences.

Calling out is often done publicly and painfully. When we are called out, we can experience intense shame and guilt. We may become defensive and dig ourselves deeper into an oppressive hole in an attempt to rationalize our ignorance and harmdoing. We may even launch a counterattack causing the exchange to spin wildly out of control. Perhaps worst of all, we may retreat to the safety of our own limited experience for fear of experiencing that shame again, removing the possibility of learning something new, of seeing something differently, of appreciating how we have choices as to whether to harm or protect others.

Sometimes the folks who do the most aggressive calling out have themselves been publicly shamed. Calling out, in this way, becomes a means of passing the buck, discharging latent shame on to another by highlighting our supposed separation: "I am the woke one; you are the ignorant harm-doer." This may in fact be true, but is it helpful? Is the objective of calling out to shame and send someone away with their tail between their legs or to raise awareness and invite someone into the realm of knowledge and compassion?

"Calling in" has been offered as an alternative. In 2013, Việt/mixed-race disabled queer writer Ngọc Loan Trân wrote on the blog *Black Girl Dangerous*:

I picture "calling in" as a practice of pulling folks back in who have strayed from us. It means extending to ourselves the reality that we will and do fuck up, we stray, and there will always be a chance for us to return. Calling in as a practice of loving each other enough to allow each other to make mistakes, a practice of loving ourselves enough to know that what we're trying to do here is a radical unlearning of everything we have been configured to believe is normal.

As mommysattvas, calling in is an essential tool in our social justice arsenal. Unlike calling out, calling in recognizes our inherent Buddha-nature. Calling in acknowledges the process of waking up, that our similarities far outweigh our differences; it is intended to be of benefit to the person who does harm as well as to all the onlookers, particularly when done publicly such as on social media. Calling in is an invitation, something clear and corrective but not shaming. Calling out may still be appropriate in some situations. It is the mommysattva's discerning wisdom that helps her know what is needed and when.

DOING OUR OWN WORK

ONLY WE KNOW where we have work to do. Books, courses, conversations, and other forms of education are indispensable, but to learn how to do better and authentically transform, we must internalize this information, feel it, process it, and practice it.

In doing our work, there are countless temptations to assuage our discomfort—performative activism, competitive wokeness, shaming others, distancing ourselves from our ignorance, emphasizing action over being with our discomfort. The real work is subtle, layered, often invisible, and not congratulated.

We are going to screw up. There is no way around that. In fact, we should be grateful for our screwups because they take us deeper; if we were to circumnavigate them, we would actually miss out on important learning. Apologizing, repairing, and doing better the next time is the path, not a detour. Doing our work requires a lot of patience and compassion. We must forgive ourselves for our ignorance while simultaneously fulfilling our obligation to overcome it.

The path and practice of meditation is inseparable from the path and practice of waking up to our own racism, sexism, ableism, ageism, transphobia, fatphobia—isms and phobias of any kind. The wisdom of our interdependence is inherent in our intrinsic enlightenment and must be not learned but uncovered.

THE FIERCE
MOTHER LINEAGE

A COMPLETE CONNECTION with the path and practice of meditation has three basic ingredients: Buddha, *dharma*, and *sangha*. The Buddha serves as an example of a human being—not to be confused with a perfect deity—who attained enlightenment. The dharma—the truth—provides the lens through which we view our day-to-day lives, helping us to meet whatever arises with the intention of waking up to reality. The sangha—the community of practitioners alone–together on this path—provides the connection and the ground we need to truly embody the teachings.

Each of us already possesses the capacity for enlightenment. To realize it, we can consume the dharma and understand it intellectually, but it is not until the dharma infuses how we interact with others that it becomes the path to enlightenment. The sangha provides us with the chance to metabolize the teachings and truly train our minds. In applying the teachings to our daily lives, we get our hands dirty, figure out what the teachings mean to us personally, challenge ourselves to step out of our safety zones, and discover the messy, beautiful, and perfectly imperfect nature of reality. It is in our engagement with the sangha that we finally see ourselves. We see where we open and where we close down, where we find comfort and where we meet our edge.

Anything I've ever done that was considered "clever" only revealed itself as such in retrospect (and by extension, anything I have done intentionally to be clever has fallen flat). I can confidently say that fumbling forward in my life, continuing to put one foot in front of the other, has been the only viable option. Many of the things I haven't felt ready to do, or felt the need to do even though I didn't completely understand why, have turned out to be life changing. Creating the Mommy Sangha was one of those things.

My son was five months old when I started to plan the Mommy Sangha and nine months old when it was officially launched. I was completely overwhelmed. The plan was to do a reading that touched on the intersections between Buddhist philosophy and motherhood, practice together, and then connect with one another. Just finding the brief reading was often too much for me, and for the first year I could be observed ten minutes before the start of our gathering frantically hunting for something relevant. But the lived experience of leading and participating in the Mommy Sangha over the past five years has been grounding, normalizing, and heart expanding. Not only did I realize that motherhood contained within it everything I needed to wake up to the truths of life, but that its constancy connected me with something that was much larger: an infinite lineage of mothers, a force to which we now belonged and with which we drive forward into the future.

For the mommysattva, the fierce mother lineage spreads out horizontally through the sangha of other moms as much as it does vertically through her biological, cultural, and spiritual heritage. In reclaiming our dignity and power as mothers, we are strengthened by the connection with all those among us and those who have come before us, with those who have transformed, sacrificed, and poured themselves into being of benefit to their own children and to the greater world of children.

The fierce mother lineage is one of compassion, lightning-strike wisdom, and a willingness to feel pain, one's own pain as well as the pain of others. It is a living, breathing, pulsing collective of individuals committed to the truth, to realizing basic goodness, and to being of benefit to others.

AN UNBROKEN LINE

IF WE TRACE THE LINE back in time—our mothers, grandmothers, great-grandmothers, and beyond—we discover the particular mother lineage that culminated in our own existence. If we are the mothers of girls, that lineage continues on, carrying with it the specific joys and sorrows experienced by each one who came before her. Each one who came before experienced matrescence, the transformation from woman to mother. She gave birth or assumed complete and primary responsibility for another human in another way, instantly transferring priority from self to child. She likely struggled with identity, felt the weight of the greatest responsibility, the fears, the pride, the need to protect. She suffered sexism, misogyny, violence, dismissal, underappreciation, and trauma. She endured suffering so that the next generation might be free of it or at least experience it in a way that might ultimately lead to awakening.

As mommysattvas, we are part of something ongoing, an unbroken line of those skilled in opening and letting go, doing what is required, and expanding to accommodate whatever arises. If we can see ourselves as part of this enormous organism, consisting of other moms and our own mother lineage, we can see more clearly how collectively we bend toward awakening, how we take all the suffering we have endured and transform it into wisdom and compassion.

COMPASSION FOR
OUR OWN MOTHERS

EVERY TIME MY OWN MOTHER SAID, "You'll understand when you have kids," I'm pretty sure I rolled my eyes. But in truth, becoming a mother has allowed me to see my own mother differently and to have compassion for her.

I can see now what she was carrying, what she struggled with, what she was able to transform, where she got stuck, how her own child-rearing was influenced by how she was raised. I can see how she tried to protect me and what she felt was most important for me to learn. I can see what she inherited and the cycles she was able to break in her own motherhood. I can see where she reached her limits, and this is where I pick up the baton.

If we are lucky, we get to see our own mothers with our children, their grandchildren. We see how that extra buffer of time and distance allows them to be different with their grandkids to how they were with us. How the distance can uncomplicate their role into one of loving unconditionally. Seeing how differently our mothers are with us and how they are with our children can crystallize where our own confusion lies, how to work with it and ultimately transform it.

Maya Angelou said, "I did then what I knew how to do. Now that I know better, I do better." The path and practice of motherhood is a steep learning curve. Our mothers did their best with what they had. In some cases, they were able to learn something new and do better. In others, not so much. Recognizing that people do the best they can allows us to forgive and to have compassion. For our own mothers and for ourselves.

BREAKING CYCLES

JUST AS WE CULTIVATE the capacity to see ourselves in real time through the practice of meditation, motherhood—the path and practice—provides us endless opportunities to see ourselves enacting habitual patterns or breaking with dysfunctional tradition and moving toward something more skillful.

Each of us inherits a legacy of pain from our mother lineage that might include abuse, neglect, violence, addiction, untreated mental illness, eating disorders, or self-loathing. Engaging with motherhood as a path gives us the opportunity to disrupt these cycles, realize the basic goodness and intelligence we all possess, and imbue the next generation with that awareness.

Each of us can only do so much. How our own mothers engaged with the path of motherhood was determined by their own upbringing, how their own mothers related to their own suffering. How our mothers excelled was largely determined by how their own mothers excelled or in direct contrast to how their own mothers fell short. Ways in which our mothers fell short were determined by other issues they were mandated to attend to. A mother might appear to not communicate self-trust to her daughter, for example, because her energy was tied up in breaking the cycle of violence she inherited from her own mother. The felt experience of lacking that self-trust is painful, but breaking the cycle of violence cannot be understated in terms of its importance to and its respect for the humanity and sovereignty of a mother's children. Another mother might resist repeating the cycle of "toughening up" her BIPOC son to prepare him for a cruel and racist world, and instead love him tenderly and unconditionally while having the brutally honest and necessary conversations she has no choice but to have with him.

When we become mothers, we inherit the karma of our mother lineage. We inherit their pain and their confusion. Their hopes and fears. The ways in which we as mothers confuse our children's stuff with our own, our own stuff with our mother's, our mother's stuff with her mother's. Meditation practice helps us see what belongs to whom, how pain and confusion are perpetuated, and how to do something different. When we can see what we have inherited directly or indirectly from our mothers, we are faced with the choice of whether harmful cycles continue down the line or stop with us.

THE MOTHER'S BODY

ONE AREA IN WHICH the mother lineage is desperately in need of reformation is in relation to the mother's body. This miraculous vessel that adapts, supports, and protects us is so often the site of aggression, criticism, and self-hatred. So many of us understandably succumb to the messaging that our bodies should be other than they are. We pathologize and fixate on some narrow slice of the whole mandala of our bodies, so that we negate what works well, what serves us so dutifully and constantly.

Our adversarial relationship with our bodies is not benign: it poisons our relationship with food, our capacity for joyful movement, our connection with our sexual and sensual selves, and our practice of basic body respect. It telegraphs to our daughters that they can find no peace in and with their bodies, that their bodies are construction sites for continual refinement. It communicates to boys that women are obligated to pursue the "best" body they could possibly have, even if that costs women joy, confidence, and self-trust, not to mention time, money, and precious limited energy. It severely stymies our capacity to find beauty everywhere.

There is an urgent need to create a new lineage of affection and reverence toward the mother's body, to blast through the walls of patriarchy and commercialism that invent problems with the mother's body only to sell them sham solutions. As activist and writer Gail Dines put it, "If tomorrow, women woke up and decided they really liked their bodies, just think how many industries would go out of business."

Instead of treating the mother's body like an ornament that must be sculpted to please the eye of the observer, mothers must be liberated to inhabit their bodies as the incredible instruments for joy, care, and positive change they are.

A LEGACY OF COMPASSION

AS MOMMYSATTVAS, we have the capacity to create a richer, subtler, and more authentic lineage that embodies kindness, feeling, searing love, and clear-seeing wisdom. We create and feed this legacy of compassion primarily through our willingness to feel pain—our own pain and the pain of others. This might sound like a hard sell but stay with me.

When we practice lovingkindness, we wish for all beings to experience safety, happiness, health, and ease from the deepest parts of our hearts. But something changes when we ourselves have experienced danger, sadness, sickness, and struggle. In drawing from our own experiences with suffering and joy and peace, and recognising the contrasts therein, lovingkindess for others takes root and blossoms in every part of our lives. Whenever we suffer, we acknowledge that suffering, feel the suffering of all who have struggled, and wish for their and our relief. When we feel joy, we acknowledge that joy, feel the collective joy of all beings, and wish to extend that experience outward.

The mother lineage that is defined by fierce compassion knows the preciousness of suffering, and that even if our natural reaction is to wish to bypass it, pain is worth staying with and exploring. Even developing friendliness for it. This practice strengthens our compassion like lifting weights can strengthen our bodies.

If increasing our capacity to tolerate discomfort is the most important skill we can develop and pass on to our children, then the mommysattva engaged in the legacy of fierce compassion is both teacher and student, master and apprentice.

WISDOM LINEAGE

JUST AS CLEAR-SEEING WISDOM, or *prajnaparamita*, is the culmination of generosity, discipline, patience, meditation, and exertion, the mother lineage is the culmination of all the mother's—all mothers'—joys, sorrows, sacrifices, realizations, pain, and satisfaction. In courageously setting forth on the path of motherhood, we live our lives colorfully and abundantly, we tangle with reality, and, ultimately, we move the needle of the populace toward full awakening.

The wisdom of mothers is hard won through experience. It is not automatic or conceptual in nature. The mother's wisdom is embodied, following the cues of her sensations and instincts, based on trial and error, and connecting with her open, living, breathing, beating heart.

THE *VAJRA* PATH

THE BUDDHA'S TEACHINGS were said to occur in three cycles: *Hinayana, Mahayana,* and *Vajrayana.* The Hinayana, or foundational vehicle, is concerned with getting your own "spiritual house" in order. It focuses on simplicity, precision, discipline, and honoring the basic precepts such as not doing harm. The Mahayana, or great vehicle, turns the practice outward to work with others. The basis for working with others are the four immeasurables of lovingkindness, compassion, sympathetic joy, and equanimity, as well as the six *paramitas* of generosity, discipline, patience, exertion, meditation, and wisdom (or *prajna*). The mommysattva practices within the teachings of the Hinayana and the Mahayana, attending both to her own spiritual awakening and to deepening that practice by clarifying her role in life to be of benefit to others.

The third cycle of the Buddha's teachings is the Vajrayana or indestructible vehicle. This cycle of teachings is connected to the sense perceptions and everyday magic. The Vajrayana teachings hold that enlightenment can happen in a snap of the fingers— that temper tantrum your child just threw, that fight with your spouse, the razor's edge between losing it or vowing to feel exactly every momentary, pulsing, raging sensation coursing through your body. In this way, the Vajra path was made for mothers: it is the fast track to enlightenment.

And if motherhood is the fast track to enlightenment, then motherhood in the pandemic was the high-occupancy-vehicle lane in the fast track. The most challenging moments, weeks, months, and years of our lives as mothers—those ages and stages that truly test our will to stay with our experience; when the cycles of closeness have diverged and we are questioning everything; the year 2020 and all its tumult, suffering, and uncertainty—these comprise the masterclass. The only way to wake up is to meet these moments directly, courageously, with the fierce open heart of the warrior mommysattva.

THE WAY OF THE MOMMYSATTVA

THE FIERCE MOTHER LINEAGE, made up of mommysattvas just like you, is always changing, pulsing, breathing in and out. The way of the mommysattva travels the concentric circles of motherhood, rippling outward and then back to where they began, like a time-lapse video showing fields of flowers reaching up out of the soil, blooming, turning toward the sun, shriveling, and ultimately dying, only to fertilize the seeds below.

The best that we can do is to live our lives. To stay awake to our own realities, our minds, hearts, and bodies. Those of our children and those of other moms. To accept ourselves as we are—warming to our imperfections, our sweetness, our best intentions—knowing that acceptance holds the potential for going beyond just the day to day.

We, the mommysattvas, explore the most personal practices of reflecting on our matrescence, working with our own mind and body, and finding the means to enlightenment in our own lives. We turn that awareness outward to include the more expansive contemplations of children as their own self-contained organisms, the inherent activism of being a mother, and being part of something larger. Then we turn it inward again to digest and discover our wisdom as it unfolds in the process of growing up and out with our children. Waves ebbing and flowing. Growing, unfolding, expanding, contracting, and coming to an end. And because we are part of something vaster, the way of the mommysattva is never really an end.

ACKNOWLEDGMENTS

THERE ARE SO MANY PEOPLE I wish to thank for supporting this project and believing in my ability to bring it to life. Susan Piver, my friend, meditation teacher, business partner, and publisher. My editor, Crystal Gandrud, who challenged and pushed me in every good way. Lisa Fehl, for always being there for a pep talk or to manage my crazy. Pema Chödrön, Jon and Myla Kabat-Zinn, Sarah Napthali, Anne Cushman, Karen Maezen Miller, and Louise Erdrich, whose books and teachings have inspired me to recognize motherhood as the path to awakening. My friends Colleen Clemens, Jennifer Teich, Sean Michael McCormick, Natisha Wallace, Shnieka Johnson, Jeanine Baisch, Mary Jane Detroyer, and Alexis Conason—you inspire me to be better. My dad, Peter; mom, Terry; sister, Melissa; brother-in-law, Jon; and nieces, Lily and Stella—I love you so, so much. Our beloved babysitter, Giovanna Cinquemani, for being my son's other mother. My partner, Andrea, for always believing in me, for never making me "too much," for growing with me, and for bringing sexy back. Mimmo, my intensitive (intense + sensitive), aggressively affectionate, wise-beyond-your-years boy—you are my heart. And the Open Heart Project Mommy Sangha members, many of whom were generous enough to share a few words, a feeling, a story, or a vignette drawn from their own experiences of motherhood to illustrate some of the more poignant points of the path for this book. We are doing it.

ABOUT THE AUTHOR

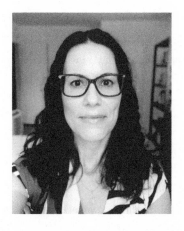

JENNA HOLLENSTEIN, MS, RDN, CDN, is a nutrition therapist, meditation teacher, and mother to Domenico. She has led the Open Heart Project Mommy Sangha (a community of moms who meditate) for five years and is the author of three books, including *Eat to Love: A Mindful Guide to Transforming Your Relationship with Food, Body, and Life*. Jenna has been featured in *Forbes, The Wall Street Journal, U.S. News & World Report, Health, Lion's Roar, mindful, Vogue, Elle, Glamour, Woman's World,* and Fox News. She lives in Mamaroneck, NY. For more information, please visit **jennahollenstein.com**.

ALSO BY LIONHEART PRESS

Lionheart Press publishes works at the intersection of spirituality and modern life. No dogma. No religion. Just deep (and deeply unconventional) thinking you won't find anywhere else.

lionheartpress.net

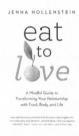

Eat to Love
A Mindful Guide to Transforming
Your Relationship with Food, Body, and Life
BY JENNA HOLLENSTEIN

"*Eat to Love* emphasizes the vital spiritual foundation of all aspects of our life—and especially our relationship to food, eating, and our bodies."

—JAN CHOZEN BAYS, MD, author of *Mindful Eating*

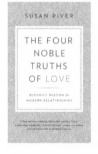

The Four Noble Truths of Love
Buddhist Wisdom for Modern Relationships
BY SUSAN PIVER

"Clear and heartwarming, this book is a guide to living relationships completely."

—SHARON SALZBERG, author of *Real Love*

CONNECT WITH LIONHEART PRESS

KEEP IN TOUCH

Join the Lionheart Press email list to find out about upcoming books and author events, teachings, or retreats. Visit **lionheart press.net** to sign up.

Join the Open Heart Project to take part in Jenna Hollenstein's Mommy Sangha and much more. Visit **openheartproject.com/ open-heart-project** to join.

SHARE YOUR PRAISE

Did you enjoy this book? Did its content and teaching benefit your life? If so, a review shared through your favorite online retailer would be warmly welcomed. A few minutes of your time may help others find this book.

PLACE A BULK ORDER

Would you like to share this book with a group or a class? Please be in touch. We offer bulk discounts for orders of ten or more copies shipped to most locations. Please write to **lisa@openheartproject.com**.

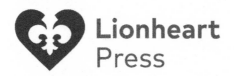

Made in the USA
Las Vegas, NV
04 September 2021

29585183R00156